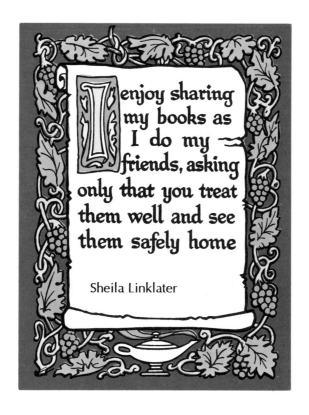

I enjoy sharing my books as I do my friends, asking only that you treat them well and see them safely home

Sheila Linklater

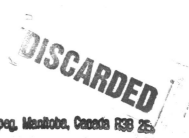

The Amazing Story of

Health Care in New China

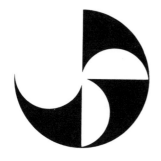

The Amazing Story of

Health Care in New China

by K. K. Jain, M.D.

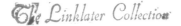

Rodale Press, Inc. Emmaus, Pa. 18049

International Standard Book Number 0-87857-072-1

Library of Congress Catalogue Number 73-7463

Copyright© 1973 by K. K. Jain

Printed in the United States of America
Printed on recycled paper

FIRST PRINTING—October, 1973
SECOND PRINTING—December, 1973
PB-287

Acknowledgements

The author wishes to thank the following for permission to quote from their publications:

1. The Journal of the Canadian Medical Association from my article "Glimpses of Chinese Medicine," Jan. 8, 1972.
2. International Surgery from my article "Neurosurgery in People's Republic of China," Feb. 1972.

Contents

Introduction

Since my days as a medical student, I have been interested in the history of medicine. Being from India, as I am, the traditional medical systems of India and China particularly fascinated me. During the past few years I have had the opportunity to travel extensively and observe present-day medical care systems in different countries. Interesting as this was, there was still a blank in my knowledge about modern China. I had some idea of the medical development in China up to the year 1964 when Dr. Wilder Penfield, the famous Montreal surgeon, wrote about China and his experiences there. But during the Cultural Revolution which followed, travel to China was very restricted and correspondence with individual physicians there was no longer possible. During this period, information about China was limited to rumors and occasional reports in the lay press.

In the latter part of 1970, Canada re-established diplomatic relations with China and the possibilities of travel to China became a reality. Early in 1971, the University of British Columbia obtained permission from the People's Republic of China to send a study group there for a one month tour. The members of the group came from different parts of Canada. I was fortunate enough to be one of them. There were Chinese scholars — Canadian teachers of Chinese from the Department of Asian studies of various universities. There were representatives of various professions; lawyers, journalists, engineers, artists and doctors. I was the representative of the practical aspects of medicine.

Before we left, most of the members of the group indicated their special interests and what places, institutions and types of activities they wanted to see. Everyone's desires were considered when the itinerary was planned. Then it was finalized by the China Travel Service, the official travel bureau of the People's Republic of China.

Our visas were issued very promptly and we flew directly to Hong Kong. After a day's stopover there we started on our journey by train to Canton. We were welcomed at the border by senior officials of the China Travel Service who had come all the way from Peking to greet us. It was then we realized that we were not classed as tourists but as guests. The Chinese frequently referred to us as a "Cultural Delegation from Canada."

The customs formalities were completed smoothly and promptly. We were pleased that we were allowed to take unlimited amounts of tapes, tape recorders, cameras, and film with us. Most of the members of our group carried their own cameras although we were given an official audio-visual recording of the tour. More than 25,000 still photographs were taken by group members. Over 18,000 feet of movie film was exposed and the combined weight of the tapes used to record sounds and conversations was over 65 pounds. We were allowed to bring this material back with us through customs without difficulty, including the undeveloped film.

During our month's stay we traveled by railway, bus, and plane, visiting major cities as well as small towns, agriculture communes, factories and hospitals. My main interest was to see the organization and practice of medicine in China and I was given many opportunities to visit hospitals and talk to Chinese physicians and health workers. It is well known by now that the Chinese allow visitors, who may not be medical men, into their operating rooms, so from time to time other members of the group joined me in visiting the hospitals and observing surgery.

I was glad that the study group I was part of represented so many different professions. It made the tour more interesting since we not only visited medical institutions but had contact with Chinese people from all walks of life and all social levels. There were frank and enlightening political discussions with groups of Chinese as well as individuals. Since some members of our group spoke fluent Chinese, we were able to communicate directly without the aid of the interpreters.

Although the tour was supervised, we were given freedom to walk anywhere on our own in the cities and villages. This sometimes created a little problem, particularly with the younger generation of Chinese who had not seen any foreigners before. Curious crowds of young people would gather, but the anxious moments eased as soon as they learned we were from Canada and came as friends.

We were very impressed by the Chinese hospitality. They were perfect hosts and treated us well at all times. We were allowed access to as much information about China as we could possibly absorb. It was an educational, eye-opening experience, both for us and for our hosts, who learned a little bit about us.

After my return, I accepted several invitations to talk about China and I wrote two papers. The public response to this information about Chinese medicine has been tremendous. People want to know more and more about it, particularly acupuncture.

This book incorporates some of my own first-hand experiences and some information imparted to me by other physicians who have visited China since 1971.

1

Centuries of Chinese Medicine

For an understanding of contemporary Chinese medicine, it is important to have some idea of its history. Chinese civilization has existed for several thousand years and its system of medicine has closely followed its philosophy of life.

I-Ching (Book of Changes) is considered the most ancient Chinese book. Basically philosophy, this book derives its name from "I" which means change. It is written in a series of hexagrams. The word "I" is used interchangeably with "Tao"—which is the spontaneous stream of life through which things are produced. All changes are considered the result of interaction between two primal forces—Yang (positive) and Yin (negative). These cosmic regulators are believed to be the basis of the entire universe. One Yin and one Yang constitutes a Tao. Though *I-Ching* is fascinating, it contains no medical information. It does, however, express the philosophy from which Chinese medicine evolved.

The most ancient medical text of China is *Huang Ti Nei Ching Su Wen, (Yellow Emperor's Classic of Internal Medicine)*. It is believed to have been written about 2,697 B.C. But the date and authorship are controversial. Some authorities state that the emperor did not have enough time to write a medical book, others disagree with the date. The English translation, by Ilza Veith, was published by the University of California Press in 1966. The book is written in the form of a dialogue between the emperor and minister, Chi Po, and contains numerous references to Taoism as well as Yin and Yang. There are many interpretations of Yang and Yin. Yang stands for sun, heavens, fine light and many related subjects. Yin stands for moon, night, cold, and so forth. Yang represents the male and Yin the female.

There is a constant interaction within the human body between Yin and Yang. The more perfectly they are balanced in a body the healthier the person is. Too much of either results in disease or death. The process of aging is due to the Yin element.

Yin and Yang are each subdivided into water, fire, metal, wood, and earth. Man was thus supposed to

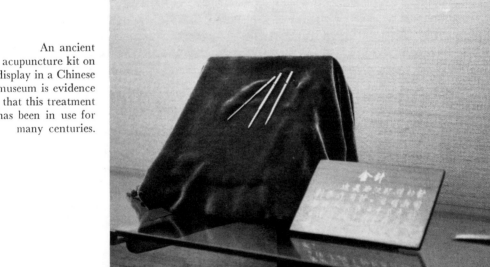

An ancient acupuncture kit on display in a Chinese museum is evidence that this treatment has been in use for many centuries.

contain these five elements in varying amounts which strengthened or weakened their Yin or Yang. The Yin-Yang principle and the five elements are also associated with the times of day and seasons of the year, for example, in spring and summer the Yin is weak and Yang dominates. The reverse is the case in winter. This theory was used to explain the seasonal variations of some diseases.

The ancient concept of Yang-Yin is still accepted in Chinese medicine and is used to explain one of the theories of acupuncture—the pulse theory.

At the time of the writing of *Yellow Emperor's Classic of Internal Medicine*, pulse diagnosis was already known. The Chinese physicians had very elaborate interpretations of various pulse rates. This was one of their main forms of diagnosis.

Acupuncture was also used at that time. It was known that various, widely-separated points all affected the function of the same organ because they were on the same meridians, called Ching. The original number of meridians was twelve, but two were added later.

The Yin-Yang principle was used in dividing internal organs into groups: passive storage organs (Yin) are lungs, spleen, heart, kidney and liver; active working organs (Yang) are large intestine, stomach, small intestine, urinary bladder and gall-bladder.

In ancient times acupuncture needles were made of flint. These were replaced by gold and silver needles, which in turn were replaced by the stainless steel needles used today. All disease was considered an imbalance between Yin and Yang. Acupuncture was aimed at restoring balance.

Surgery was seldom used in ancient Chinese society, although skulls found during excavations reveal that trepanation (drilling through the skull) operations were practiced thousands of years ago in China.

A few hundred years before Christ the Chinese and the Indians exchanged medical information. Of particular interest are the Buddhist translations of important Indian medical works into Chinese, such as *Charak, (Textbook of Medicine)* and *Sushruta (Textbook of Surgery)*. The Chinese borrowed some of the herbal remedies from the Indian system of medicine, but for some unknown reasons acupuncture was never introduced into India. The Chinese adapted very little of the Indian system of surgery although it was the most highly-developed of any ancient form of surgery.

Greek civilization also influenced Chinese medicine to some extent. Pien Ch'ueh, "father of the pulse," was a contemporary of the famous Greek physician Hippocrates. During this period, there were Chinese works on prescriptions, physical culture, respiratory techniques, and the study of sex. Chang Chung-Ching, the Chinese Hippocrates, who was born around 158 B.C., was the first to codify the Chinese symptomatology and therapeutics and also the first to differentiate clearly between Yin and Yang symptoms. He compiled authoritative works entitled *Shang-han-lun (Treatise of Ailments Caused by Cold)* which is still used by the traditional Chinese physicians.

Yuan Hua (also called Hua T'o) was a great surgeon of this period. His most important medical contributions were in the field of anaesthetics (using Indian hemp, Ma-fi-san) and abdominal operations. The first operations involving grafting of organs and thoracotomies (surgical incision of the chest cavity) are credited to him, but this is difficult to accept as there were no adequate surgical instruments at the time. Yuan Hua is also reputed to have cured the violent headaches of Emperor Ts'ao Ts'ao of Northern China by using acupuncture. At a later date he suggested skull trepanation to cure another illness of the ailing emperor. Unfortunately for Yuan Hua, the emperor didn't take kindly to this suggestion. He had Yuan-Hua imprisoned and in the year 208 A.D. ordered his execution. In an effort to preserve his writings Yuan-Hua entrusted them to his jailor but the man was so frightened of punishment that he burned the manuscripts. Somehow Yuan-Hua's *Treatise on Medicine* survived and was printed as late as 960. Many of the anatomical charts he drew which showed the inside of the human body are still in existence today.

The Han period (206 B.C. to 220 A.D.) is considered an important era in Chinese medicine. Both Chung-Ching and Hua T'o lived during this period. Other eminent medical men were Huang-Fu Mi (215-282) author of a classical work on acupuncture and Wang Shu-ho (265-317) whose writings on the pulse, which were translated into several Western languages, were used up to the 18th century.

The great period of Taoism stretched from the third century B.C. to the seventh century A.D. Ko Hung (281-340) one of the most notable Taoist alchemists wrote two important medical works, *The Medication in the Golden Box* and *First Aid Measures*. He had a clear idea of preventive medicine and was the first one to describe smallpox (five centuries before Arabian Rhazes). Many of his teachings have survived through the ages and their influence is seen in modern China. His advice for longevity "rising at cock's crow and ending activities at sunset," is still followed by millions of Chinese. And respiratory exercises, which he also claimed promoted long life, are widely-practiced in China today.

Ko Hung was the first person to describe symptoms of tuberculosis, beri-beri, hepatitis and bubonic plague. He also produced works on therapeutics—prescribing cheap, easily-available herbs—but very few of them are still in use.

Forensic medicine (the branch of medicine dealing with crime and law) did not earn its status as a specialty until the publication of *Hsi Yuan Li (Instructions to Coroners)*. This was compiled in 1247 at a time when Europe had no analogous books. This comprehensive text on legal medicine was used by magistrates and coroners. The principles of the book are portrayed in a watercolor painting entitled *An Inquest in Old China,* which shows a magistrate, seated on a horse and shaded by an umbrella, presiding over an autopsy. The coroner assisted by two apprentices is examining a corpse. One of the apprentices holds an oiled, silk umbrella in such a manner that filtered sunlight falls on the area being examined. This prevention of glare allows stains and bruises to be seen better. The second apprentice is grinding a mixture of onions, red pepper, salt, white prunes, grain mash, and vinegar to make a hot paste. This is to be spread on parts of the body to bring out wounds by its drying action. Also present in the scene are a recording official to write down the coroner's observations and a surveyor to fix the exact location of the body.

This book was in use as late as 1924. Its introduction states that one of the reasons for *post-mortem* examination is to confirm the validity of statements in a confession, thus preventing rich criminals from paying substitutes to falsely confess to crimes. The work is considered a masterpiece of medical jurisprudence, although the Chinese Academy of Medicine no longer approves of it as a textbook. Actual *post-mortem* examinations were limited, due to Confucian belief in the sacredness of the body. A law to facilitate the dissection of dead bodies was not passed in China until 1913.

During the Ming Dynasty (1368-1644) there were further advances in Chinese medicine. The masterpiece of this period was *Materia Medica of Li-Shih-Chen*

(1518-1593). This was translated into all of the Far Eastern languages and later into the principal Western languages. The great compendium of remedies documented 12,000 prescriptions and formulas—analyzed 1,074 plant substances, 443 animal substances, and 354 mineral substances. According to this book, syphilis appeared in China around 1505, during the same time it was detected in Europe.

The Ch'ing Dynasty (1644-1911) brought foreign rule to China again. During this time great encyclopedic works were published by Imperial Commissions. These included large medical sections. China did not become acquainted with Western medicine until the first Opium War (1839-1842). Western medicine was not very popular at first, but it became more widely-accepted after the People's Revolution (1911). At this time, many Western doctors visited China. Some of them were so impressed with the country that they settled down and established practices there.

Among the Canadian doctors in China was Dr. Omar Leslie Kilborn who went there in 1891 as a missionary doctor. He was among the international group of medical missionaries who founded the Faculty of Medicine at West China Union University in Chengtu, in 1914. In addition to medicine, he taught basic subjects such as physics and chemistry. Dr. Kilborn and his doctor wife, who helped him in his work, lived through some very turbulent times in Chinese history. During the Chinese revolution of 1911, he helped organize the Chinese Red Cross. Leaving the comforts of a well-equipped modern hospital, Dr. Kilborn worked under primitive conditions, walking barefoot through mud, to serve the sick and wounded. When he died of pneumonia in 1920, his wife carried on his work for the next twelve years. Later, their doctor-son taught at the same medical school.

In 1937, when the Sino-Japanese war erupted, universities from northern and eastern China sought refuge in Chengtu. Following in his father's footsteps, Dr. Kilborn, with the aid of his wife, undertook the almost superhuman task of accommodating the refugee universities. When the Japanese bombed Chengtu in 1939, the Kilborns moved to Jenshow and remained there until the end of the war.

In 1943, when Canada and China first reestablished diplomatic relations, Dr. Kilborn was requested by the Canadian government to assist the newly appointed Canadian ambassador to China, General Victor Odlum. After World War II the refugee universities moved out of Chengtu but life at Western China Union University had barely returned to normal before it was disrupted by the Civil War. Chengtu was occupied by the liberation army of Mao-Tse-Tung in 1949. In 1952 the Kilborns left Chengtu after years of dedicated service to China.

China was a National Republic from 1912-1949 and the influence of Western medicine increased. In 1913, the Rockefeller Foundation established the Peking Union Medical College. The first medical students were enrolled in 1919. At one time, it was considered one of the leading medical schools in the world. Graduates became leaders of medicine and public health under the Kuomintang government. Around 1935, there were thirty-three faculties of medicine and five hundred hospitals in China and approximately 18,000 doctors practiced Western medicine. This number kept increasing until the Japanese invasion in 1940.

One of the best known American doctors practicing in China during those days (and he is still there) was Dr. George Hatam, known to the Chinese as Dr. Ma (referred to as Dr. Horse by Edgar Snow in his book "Red China Today"). Born in Buffalo, New York in 1910 of

Syrian parents, he studied medicine in Switzerland. In 1933, he and two other American doctors studying in Geneva decided to set up practices in China. He started in Shanghai and his practice in venereal diseases flourished. Dr. Hatam was discouraged with corruption in Shanghai and felt that treating V.D. patients was futile as long as organized crime promoted prostitution.

In 1936 he crossed over to the communist territory and met Mao-Tse-Tung. While there, he married a Chinese girl, and from then on worked for the people but he continued to take a special interest in the control of venereal diseases. After the liberation of Shanghai in 1949 he took a leading part in the eradication of venereal disease in that city. Later he moved to Peking and became deputy director of the Institute of Venereology. During the Cultural Revolution this institute was moved out of the city, but Dr. Ma still lives and works in Peking. It is of interest that he still retains his American citizenship.

By the time of liberation in 1949, there were from 20,000 to 45,000 Western type doctors in China with a ratio of about one doctor for every 25,000 people. In the United States at that time the physician population ratio was 1 to 750. When the Communist Government took over there were great improvements made in the medical care system, and parasitic and venereal diseases were almost wiped out. A good account of those days is given by a well-known British surgeon, J. S. Horn, who went to China in 1954. His autobiography "Away With All Pests" was published in 1969 and gives a personal account of his experiences in China. He saw many sick, neglected people—the legacy of almost total medical neglect of the laboring class before liberation. Among the things which dismayed him were cases of dislocated joints which had remained unreduced for ten years or more.

Dr. Horn had a humiliating experience when he removed the spleen of a patient who had a bleeding disorder. The patient did not improve and a traditional Chinese doctor cured the patient with a single dose of an herbal potion. Dr. Horn humbly admits that he learned many things from the patients and saw rare diseases that he had not encountered in England.

Over the following fourteen years, he did tremendous amounts of general surgical work, although he was primarily a specialist in diseases of the bones and joints. He adapted to the Chinese way of life and learned to respect the social customs. The informal relationship between patient and doctors based on equality and mutual respect impressed him greatly. In 1969, just when the Cultural Revolution was starting, he left China to return to England and teach Orthopedic Surgery. I had an opportunity to attend a public lecture he delivered in Auckland (N.Z.) on August 17, 1972. He stated firmly that China is the only country where venereal diseases have been wiped out. He said he left China because he felt there were enough well-trained Chinese doctors and he was no longer needed.

Around the time of the liberation many European physicians, who practiced in China, went back to Europe where they introduced acupuncture into their practices. It still flourishes today.

After the liberation of China the Russians also came along to help in the reconstruction. They sent some of their leading medical specialists, including the famous Russian neurosurgeon Arutnow, who helped organize a neurosurgical training program in Peking. However, the Russians split with China over ideologic matters, and most of the Russian physicians had left China by 1960, taking a knowledge of acupuncture back to Russia. There are still occasional publications in Russian literature on acupuncture, but they did not adopt it on any significant scale.

Traditional medicine suffered a set-back in 1912. From then until 1949 only about eight institutions of traditional medicine were allowed to operate. The practitioners of traditional medicine were looked upon as charlatans. After the liberation, in 1949, interest in traditional medicine was renewed, and in 1968 the Cultural Revolution led to the merger of Western and traditional medicine.

2

Western Medicine and Traditional Chinese Medicine Join Forces

In 1966, the second revolution, called "The Great Proletarian Cultural Revolution," started in China. It continued for the next three years. This revolution affected all facets of Chinese life including education and medicine. Directions given by Chairman Mao Tse-tung, were carried out by students and so-called "Red Guards." Some of the powerful academic and professional leaders were deposed and "encouraged" to readjust to the new society.

The following quotation is from "Official Documents of the Great Proletarian Cultural Revolution in China" (Peking Foreign Language Press 1970, p.149, Item No. 10, Educational Reform)—"In the Great Cultural Revolution the most important task is to transform the old educational system and the old principles and methods of teaching.

"In this Great Cultural Revolution the phenomena of our schools being dominated by bourgeois intellectuals must be completely changed.

"In every kind of school we must apply thoroughly the policy advanced by Comrade Mao Tse-tung of Education serving Proletarian Politics and the Proletarian Politics and Education being combined with productive labor, so as to enable those receiving an education to develop morally, intellectually, and physically, and to become laborers with socialistic consciousness and culture.

"The period of schooling should be shortened. The courses should be fewer and better. The teaching materials should be thoroughly transformed, in some cases beginning with simplifying complicated material. While their main task is to study, students should also learn other things. That is to say, in addition to their studies, they should also learn industrial work, foreign and military affairs, and take part in the struggles of the Cultural Revolution to criticize the bourgeoisie as these struggles occur."

It is apparent that there were strong political overtones in the medical developments. During the Cultural Revolution, all the medical schools were closed. But a few medical students, who had already enrolled, were allowed to finish their educations in hospitals. There was practically no contact with Western medicine. Few Western physicians entered China and no Chinese physicans were permitted to visit Western countries. No research was done and no medical literature was published during this period as this type of work was viewed by the government as "self-glorification." The doctors did not hold any meetings, express any opinions, or write any textbooks for fear of criticism. The famous *Chinese Medical Journal* ceased publication in 1968 and has not yet resumed. But the greatest change in the medical scene was the merger of Western and traditional Chinese medicine. The practitioners of Chinese medicine were no longer looked down upon as quacks or second-rate physicians. They were upgraded to a respectable position in society and given an opportunity to learn Western medicine. Similarly, doctors of Western medicine were encouraged to study traditional medicine.

The result of this merger was a large medical force able to cope with the needs of the teeming millions. It also improved the standard of medical care. The combination of Western and Chinese medicine produced some remarkable innovations such as acupuncture anaesthesia which will be discussed in a later chapter.

In China, 90 percent of the people live in rural areas. In order to bring top professionals closer to the masses, there was a movement of doctors, particularly specialists, from the big cities to the countryside. Most of these moves were a reaction to Mao's directive, "Medical and Health Work," which put the stress on rural areas.

This was the greatest benefit derived from the change. A large segment of the population who lived in the villages got medical treatment. There were many people who prior to liberation (1949) received no medical aid. After the liberation, their medical care was mostly traditional Chinese medicine. Since the second revolution, the peasants get the best possible medical care, if not in their own country hospital, then in the big city hospital to which they are transferred and looked after by the most qualified physicians available. While visiting various hospitals I had occasion to ask the patients how they felt. They always prefaced their statements by saying: "Thanks to Chairman Mao I am very well looked after." These patients are probably right. Prior to the liberation they would not have even dreamed of being brought into a modern hospital to receive the latest treatment from skilled specialists.

How the physicians were affected by the Cultural Revolution is best illustrated by interviews with the Chi-

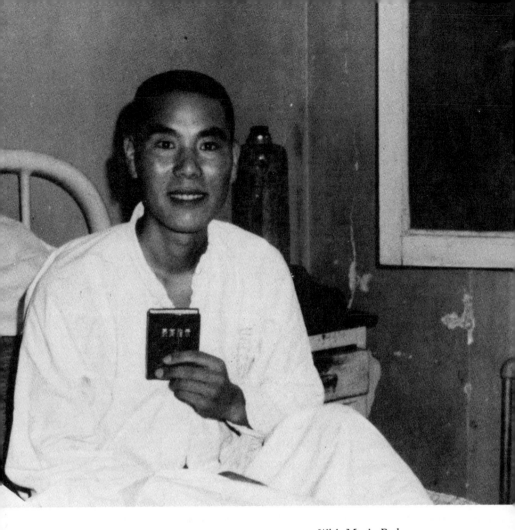

With Mao's *Red Book* in hand, a patient in a Chinese hospital greets visitors.

nese doctors. The first one I talked to was Dr. K. L. Yang, Professor of Dermatology, Shanghai Medical University: "I lived in the old society for fifty years. I used to sit in the office, direct others and never go to the masses. During the revolution I studied Chairman Mao's writings and improved my ideology. Though I had been a party member for ten years, my outlook was still old. In order to change my old outlook, I went to the countryside to change my thinking. In October 1968, I joined a Workers' Team and learned from them. I went to a commune and slept on a wooden bed with only a mat on it. This was the first time I had used such a bed. Mao teaches that a communist should try to correct every difficulty that he encounters. After one week I got used to it.

"In my work, I had to climb mountains. Other comrades told me that I was too old and should not climb mountains. I reminded myself that I should go to the place that is most difficult. I started at the lower mountain and then the ones more than 100 meters high. I had some palpitation and shortness of breath but I gradually adapted to this.

"The most significant change in my work style occurred in this manner. In the past, I was teaching and treating patients, not for rendering service to the people but to collect material for writing books and papers. Now I look at my work as a servant of the people. I also do some physical labor with the masses. In the past, I was a bourgeois specialist and this is a new beginning for me. In comparison with Comrade Bethune* I felt I was way behind. I went to Peking in 1969 and met Chairman Mao and came back to Shanghai. I was advised to retire as I was over seventy years of age. I refused. Now I am back

---

*Dr. Norman Bethune—a Canadian surgeon who served with Mao Tse-tung's Army during the struggle for liberation. Dr. Bethune is a hero to the Chinese people.

in scientific work and my work is more related to practice. Take, for example, the treatment of eczema. In the past we treated patients with medicines, but now we try to mobilize the patient's own defenses and try to remove the irritants."

The next interview was with Dr. Kuo Shusu. This was in response to my request to meet a neurologist in Tsinan. Dr. Shusu, who was wearing an army uniform, came from the People's Liberation Army Hospital. He was introduced as a "Nerve Doctor." He appeared to be neither a psychiatrist nor a neurologist. His statement is reported verbatim:

"I am a very ordinary doctor in the hospital. I have not studied Mao's work very well and I have much work to do. Particularly, my ideological work is not well done. We have achieved some success in our work because we have correct leadership at our hospital. I have done some work in curing common nerve diseases." He then talked about his ideological reformation. "I entered the Army at the age of fifteen. I was a boy medical worker and received only five years education in a primary school. I learned medical work on the battlefield. I had only one desire, and that was to cure diseases. In 1957, The Party sent me to a medical university and I went through five years of medical education, but at the end I felt my ability was reduced. I did not have the same spirit for identifying with a patient as I had when working as a soldier. I was sent to another medical institute to specialize in nerve medicine for two years. I buried my head in books and had 1,005 pieces of notes. It is so funny that my medical knowledge increased but my ability to cure went down. I was getting worried about myself. Then, according to Chairman Mao's instructions in 1965, I joined a medical mobile team. I went to live with soldiers and found that I had regained the feeling of identifying with the people."

Life of a Chinese Doctor

Prior to the liberation of China there were many different categories of doctors. The European doctors practicing in big cities had a rich clientele. They lived like aristocrats in mansions staffed with many Chinese servants. In contrast, the traditional Chinese doctor did not have any more status than an average businessman. In 1949, the foreign doctors left, but the class structure persists among the Chinese physicians. The specialists trained in Western medicine still have higher positions and are paid far more than ordinary doctors. Even the Cultural Revolution did not change the disparity in their incomes. A professor in a medical school gets five to six times the salary of a beginning general physician.

I did not have the opportunity to visit the homes of any Chinese physicians. To my knowledge neither did any of the other visiting North American physicians. Most of our meetings were in public places or in hospitals. This made it difficult to observe the personal life of a Chinese physician. So the following comments have to be evaluated in the light of this limitation.

The doctors dress very informally, no different from office workers or travel guides. Their housing is equivalent to that of other members of the society in the area in which they live. Country doctors live very much like farmers in similar types of cottages. Since no private citizens in China have cars, the doctors usually ride bicycles to work. In rural areas where there are no suitable roads, they sometimes ride donkeys to make house calls.

Fixed hours of work enable the Chinese doctors to spend more time with their families than the Western doctors can. Chinese doctors often marry medical workers, nurses, or lady doctors, and in this situation both husband and wife work. There are no private clubs to which these physicians belong, and they don't appear to have many hobbies. The opportunities for travel are very limited and are usually professional. There was a physician who accompanied us on the portions of our trip which took us away from populated areas and medical centers. His job was to provide medical aid in case of the illness of a member of our group. He was happy to have the opportunity to travel and meet foreigners and he was curious about the life of a Western doctor. The high income of Western physicians and our independent way of life amazed him. But he appeared to be well adjusted and happy in his work.

Chinese physicians don't have any higher incidence of mental illness or gastric ulcers than the general population. This cannot be said for Western doctors who suffer greatly from stress. I did not meet any Chinese physician who was overworked or under great stress.

The Chinese doctor doesn't enjoy a particularly prominent position in society. The politician is far more important, even in the hospital setting. The Chinese specialist who devises a new procedure gains eminence in his field, but is never given much publicity as an individual. Credit goes to the new political system and the doctor remains in the background. There are no financial rewards, medals of honor or titles for doctors. It is even difficult to locate the name of the doctor who first administered acupuncture anaesthesia.

Travel abroad is almost non-existent among Chinese doctors. Only a handful of Chinese have visited Canada in the last year. Possibly more will come to Canada and the United States in the next year and we may have the opportunity to learn about their lives and their feelings.

Contrast this to the doctor in North America. He belongs to the elite group of society, usually lives in an expensive house, owns a late-model car, a yacht, or even a private airplane. He dresses well and so does his wife. Doctors are among the highest earning professional people in North America.

A specialist in North America who devises a new procedure, or gains some prominence in his field, gets a lot of publicity (although it is still considered a little bit unethical). To be written up in *Time* magazine or even the local newspaper is a milestone in a specialist's life. With fame comes fortune and the opportunity to travel, attending conventions.

I personally think that the only people who go into medicine in China today are those who are strongly motivated towards serving people. In Western society status and financial rewards are often prominent reasons for selecting medicine as a career. Most of the younger Chinese physicians have a humble heritage. Some of them were soldiers or farmers before becoming doctors and they are close to the people they serve. Physicians in North America generally come from well-to-do families and often have little in common with their patients.

3

China's
Medical Machine

Administration

The Chinese Ministry of Health is located in Peking. It has five main departments:

1. Public Health

2. Medical Education

3. Medical Services—Hospitals and Clinics

4. Child and Maternal Medicine

5. Medical Supplies—Manufacture, Import and Export of Drugs, plus Hospital Equipment

All health policies are determined by the ministry and carried out by the twenty-one provinces (excluding Taiwan), five autonomous districts, (national minorities) plus three autonomous cities—Peking, Shanghai, and

Tientsin. For administrative purposes, each province is divided into 2,000 counties. Each county medical service administers to clinics and hospitals in 15-20 communes. Each commune, which is an economic unit of the county, consists of 40-50 brigades.

Medical Economics

The medical services are financed with revenue received by the government from the following sources:

1. Income from national enterprises, such as industry or department stores. Most of the major enterprises are controlled by the State.

2. Agricultural tax—paid by the communes. This is usually paid in kind, e.g. agricultural products such as rice to contribute to national food stockpile.

3. Customs—duties. (There is no sales tax, however.)

4. Labor insurance. This is paid by the factories for all workers.

5. Premiums for medical insurance. The government contributes this for its employees, but their families have to pay half of the usual premium rates. In case of peasants, the premium is paid by the communes and is regarded as a charge against running their commune. These premiums are quite nominal and would equate with taking about a dollar a month from the average Western income. The insurance covers medical care, drugs, and hospitalization. (The People's Liberation Army runs a small hospital where soldiers are treated free, but they also accept civilian patients).

It may be added that there is no income tax in China.

In the Province of British Columbia, the sales tax is supposed to cover hospitalization expenses. Patients pay $5.00 per month for coverage of medical services. They pay a nominal charge of $1.00 per day to stay in the hospital. An average Canadian contributes about the same percentage of his income to medical coverage as a Chinese. But other things, like rent and food, are more expensive in Canada and the United States, so the Chinese with a small income still has a larger percentage of his earnings left.

Medical Manpower

The exact number of medical personnel in China is as indefinite as the total population of China which has been estimated between 700,000,000 and 800,000,000. There are no statistics available so I have used only approximate figures.

The various categories of medical workers are not clearly defined. The term "M.D." is not used in the same sense as we apply it. Generally speaking, the following categories are recognized but they overlap:

1. Doctors originally trained in Western medicine with training in traditional Chinese medicine

2. Doctors originally trained in traditional Chinese medicine with training in Western medicine

3. Medical students

4. Barefoot doctors, worker doctors, or Red Guard doctors

5. Nurses

6. Acupuncturists

7. Public health workers

8. Pharmacists

9. Midwives

10. Part-time medical workers and non-medical political workers in medical organizations

11. Medical technicians (x-ray technicians, lab technicians, etc.)

In North America, there are many categories of medical workers too:

1. The M.D.'s or the doctors trained in the Western system of medicine predominate. We base our figures of doctor to population ratio on these doctors. Their number is well determined and up-to-date figures are available.

2. Doctors in other healing arts, such as osteopathy, naturopathy, chiropractic and homeopathy, constitute a significant health workers' force, particularly in the United States. There is no corresponding category of physicians in China.

3. Medical students in North America could be equated to the medical students in China with two basic differences. First, there is a much larger number of them in North America. We have approximately one hundred medical schools with classes varying anywhere from fifty to one hundred students. In China, the number of students is very

small. Second, Chinese medical students work in the countryside while they are learning and they constitute an important part of China's health team. In North America few medical students work as part of their study.

4. There are a growing number of medical assistants. These people are not trained as doctors, but are knowledgeable in minor medical procedures and are valuable in aiding physicians. There is a category of these workers called "Medex." This word, of French derivation, means medicine-extension. It is applied in the United States to ex-military corpsmen who served in Vietnam and are proficient in handling trauma. After a few months' training, following discharge from the army, they are of great help to doctors. Canada is attempting to develop a Medex Corps from their existing nursing staff.

5. In North America, there is about one nurse for every 250 persons, whereas in China, there are very few nurses.

6. Our Public Health workers are comparable to those in China.

7. Pharmacists are basically the same.

8. We still have midwives. Though their number is rather small, the ancient art is becoming popular again.

9. Medical technicians, such as x-ray technicians and laboratory workers.

10. We do not have any medical political workers.

11. There are a handful of acupuncturists and practitioners of Chinese medicine in North America.

Prior to the Cultural Revolution in China, the services of the 100,000 practitioners of Western medicine and the 600,000 practitioners of Chinese medicine were not being adequately utilized. They are now being used more efficiently and, in addition, there are nearly 1,000,000 acupuncturists, at least 150,000 of these are physicians. One million barefoot doctors, over 3,000,000 part-time health workers, 200,000 nurses, 50,000 midwives, about 100,000 pharmacists and an undetermined number of medical students complete China's medical force.

It is difficult to compare the health manpower situation in China with that of North America. Many factors such as activity of physicians, type of ailment and differences in the roles of the health workers determine the quality of care. We have a much larger professionally trained health force than the Chinese but, in terms of effective delivery to the common man, perhaps the Chinese are doing better. There are many people in the United States who do not get good medical care because of their geographic location or economic situation. In China, a person in an outlying rural community gets the same high-quality medical care as a person living in a big city. The poorer members of the Chinese society receive medical treatment equal to that of the higher classes.

The Doctors

Some of China's medical doctors were trained in Western medical schools in China and some in schools abroad, prior to liberation. Since the Cultural Revolution, most of these doctors have had some training in Chinese medicine. During the Cultural Revolution some of the professors of Western medicine spent a few months in the countryside, but most of them returned to their original positions. They work in close collaboration with the traditional Chinese physicians—often in the same institution.

Although most of the physicians are male, the number of female doctors is increasing. Most of the physicians belong to the Chinese Medical Association which holds the authority previously vested in the Chinese Academy of Medical Science. This is not a political union, but an association for dissemination of information. As yet they have not held any meetings, but have invited and acted as hosts for foreign physicians.

It is difficult to compare the Chinese Medical Association with the American Medical Association. The American Medical Association is a very well-organized society with a much larger number of physicians. It wields a lot of political power and maintains a lobby in Washington. Its members are deeply involved in determining medical morality, medical-legality and medical journalistic practices. By comparison, the Chinese Medical Association is inactive.

All doctors in China are state employees. They have fixed hours of work—usually 7:00 a.m. to 11:00 a.m. and 1:30 p.m. to 3:30 p.m. Outside these hours, emergency calls are taken on a rotating system. The lowest salary for a young doctor is 60 yuan per month (1 yuan is equal to 40¢). The average salary is about 90 yuan per month. In the field of education, a deputy professor gets from 160 to 200 yuan per month and a first grade professor gets up to 360 yuan per month. These salary scales have remained unchanged from those prior to the Cultural Revolution. I asked my hosts about the disparity and was told that efforts are being made to equalize the salary scales. Some highly-paid professors have voluntarily cut down their salaries, but this has not been enforced by the State. The usual retirement age for male doctors is sixty and for female doctors fifty-five. Pensions vary according to the length of service and are usually 70 percent to 80 percent of the salary at the time of retirement. A doctor may, however, voluntarily continue to work on a consultant basis after he is retired.

The salary of a first rate doctor is equivalent to about $150 per month. This is considered a great deal in China where there is no such thing as inflation or the shrinking value of the dollar. Clothing is quite inexpensive because the people dress modestly and housing is cheap—a few dollars at most pays rent for a month. The cost of premiums for medical care is quite small. Food costs little. For instance, meat is about 75¢ per pound, fish only about 30¢ per pound and eggs are about 3¢ per dozen. There are no travel expenses and the doctors do not buy any expensive books or journals. Nor do they have to own any of their own private equipment. There is a lot of money left over for savings, even at a salary of $150 per month.

The Chinese are allowed to have private bank accounts and some of them do save money. From time to time they indulge in buying some personal item of luxury such as a wrist watch or a radio. These are rather expensive, but still priced lower than their counterpart products in the West. A good Chinese-made camera costs around $100.

Most doctors of traditional medicine avail themselves of the opportunity to study Western medicine. But they still emphasize the Chinese way of treating with herbs and acupuncture. Although they have their own departments in hospitals, they treat patients in close cooperation with the Western type of physicians. A typical

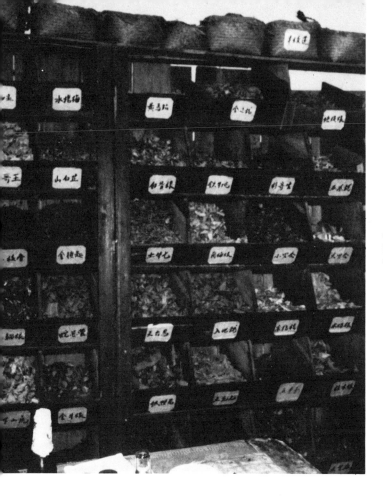

A well-stocked herbal pharmacy in a commune hospital.

This computer-type apparatus speeds up the process of compounding herbal prescriptions.

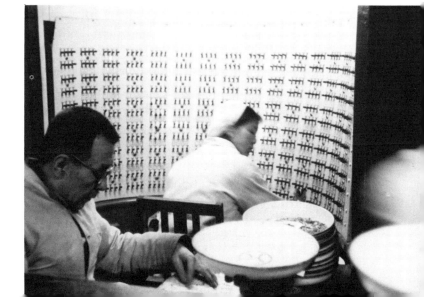

example is that of a patient with appendicitis. He will first be treated with herbs, but if he does not improve he will be operated on by a surgeon from a group of doctors who are basically trained in Western medicine.

It is difficult to evaluate the efficiency of herbal medicines in treating appendicitis as there are not enough controlled statistics available. We know that some patients with appendicitis improve on their own, but it is an inflammatory ailment and it is conceivable that the herbs may reduce the inflammation. This is difficult to prove. If a patient has surgery for appendicitis, the diagnosis is confirmed by post-operative examination of the appendix. But if a patient improves on herbal medication, it raises the question of whether the patient had appendicitis in the first place. However, it appears to be a reasonable approach to try medication first, while the patient is observed by a surgeon. Then, if there is any sign of deterioration, the appendix can be removed. One of the major dangers in appendicitis is a rupture of the appendix. This is the only major objection to trying medical treatment first and delaying surgery in the case of acute appendicitis.

The Chinese are trying herbal medications in almost all acute inflammatory conditions, including gallbladder inflammations. There is the additional use of herbs as antibiotics for infections such as lung abscesses or pneumonia. When the treatment of abscesses has been successful the need for involved surgery to allow drainage has been eliminated. But statistics are not available for analysis by the Western physicians. The fact that herbs cure some diseases previously treated by surgery is not surprising. In the past, many of the so called "wonder drugs" have been made from herbs. Surpasil, which is used for treatment of hypertension, is a good example of this. In ancient Indian herbal medicine, it was used for treatment of high blood pressure under the name of

Rauwfola Serpentina. Some of these herbs which help infection may be endowed with properties similar to antibiotics.

Barefoot Doctors

Barefoot doctors (named for the peasants of Southern China who work barefoot in the rice paddies) are defined as "peasants who have had basic medical training and give treatment without leaving productive work." All the barefoot doctors that I spoke to were wearing shoes. These much-talked-about health workers are addressed by the people as "comrades" to distinguish them from regularly trained doctors. The counterpart of a barefoot doctor in a factory is a worker doctor.

The Red Guard doctor is usually a housewife, who has been given ten days of medical training. The Red Guard doctors from neighboring units meet once a week for lectures and to exchange experiences. Their major role is in prevention of disease and they are also responsible for immunization and dispersing birth control information.

Though most of these Red Guard doctors are young housewives, there is nothing unusual about them socially. Their work is quite effective because they are known in their neighborhoods and they work gratis. But they are more politically indoctrinated than worker doctors or barefoot doctors.

Most barefoot doctors are high school graduates with three to six months training in medical work. Some of them are selected, by their communities, to become doctors and then return to work in their communes. They evolved out of medical needs for rural China. Because 80-percent of the population of China lives in villages they had very little medical aid prior to the liberation.

Partly modeled after the Russian Feldshers (physicians' assistants) of the late 1950's, the barefoot doctors' duties vary according to the area but first aid, sanitation, and immunization are generally included. Their salaries are close to that of a peasant (25 yuan a month).

The *Barefoot Doctor Manual* is standard equipment. It contains basic medical information and first aid directions. Herbs, simple medications—such as aspirin, antibiotics, tranquilizers, bandages, acupuncture needles, and a thermometer can be found in the medical bag of every barefoot doctor. These doctors are particularly knowledgeable about herbs and acupuncture.

If someone living on a farm has a stomach ache, he is treated first by the barefoot doctor. If the patient does not have relief, he is transferred to the commune hospital. The barefoot doctor usually accompanies the patient to the hospital. But 80 to 85 percent of these patients are relieved of their minor ailments without hospitalization.

One barefoot doctor I met was a twenty-three year old girl who had a high school education and six months medical training. She works on a farm most of the time, and spends about four hours a day on medical work. She told me how she saved a peasant's life by correctly applying a tourniquet after a leg injury. Some day she would like to be a physician.

The barefoot doctor concept is of great interest to North American physicians. It would compensate for the shortage of doctors in remote areas of the United States and Canada. It would also relieve the overworked general practitioner who has to handle many minor problems which do not require a fully trained physician.

Under the present circumstances, it is difficult to induce physicians to set up practices in remote areas.

People living in these areas could benefit enormously even from a medical worker with only basic medical knowledge.

Nurses

Nurses are in short supply in China. Although they rarely work in hospital wards the patients are well cared for. The Chinese patients generally require less nursing care because they help each other and ambulatory patients make their own beds and go to the cafeteria for meals. They sometimes prepare their own medications and in one hospital were assisting in the manufacture of drugs from herbs. The nurses have few non-clinical responsibilities. Most of their time is spent caring for patients who can't care for themselves.

Although we have more nurses in North America, the patient care is not necessarily better. The nurses are required to waste a lot of their time on clerical work and other non-clinical tasks. The nurses' responsibilities vary in different hospitals, and in some situations they are not allowed to handle simple medical matters without consulting the doctors. This wastes the nurses' time as well as the doctors'. Common examples of this are changing bandages and dressings for surgical patients and ordering simple medication for relief of pain. Giving intravenous medications is another thing that nurses are competent to do but they are not allowed to in most hospitals.

Some of the private patients in our hospitals live like they would in a hotel. The nurses act as waiters, bringing their food trays to them. Many of these patients could get up and help themselves if proper dining facilities were available. Some hospitals are creating ambulatory wards of patients who are well enough to feed and dress themselves. This lessens the amount of work for the nurses. In our system of medicine, the nurse still plays a vital role. But if she were relieved of her unnecessary tasks, she could take more responsibility for individual management of patients. Our nurses are not allowed to tell patients the results of any tests. I feel that they could be a vital link in the communication of medical information from doctor to patient.

In our system, it is very difficult for a nurse to further her study of medicine. She must go to a college for the premedical requirements, then complete medical school.

Nurses in China generally start training at the age of sixteen after graduating from middle school (the four years after five years of primary school). The usual training period is three years. After the first two, they take on the full duties of a graduate nurse. There are no examinations. They do not receive any salary during their training, but during the first year after graduation they are paid 40 yuan per month. The average salary of a nurse is 60 yuan per month but matrons get as much as 120 yuan per month ($50.00 US). The nurses are close to doctors in status as well as salary. In the care of a patient, the nurse is a member of a team. She has an equal say in deciding the course of treatment. The patient also has an equal voice in deciding his treatment once he has been briefed on his condition and the possible courses of action.

Nurses in China often assist doctors in the operating room in major surgical procedures and some nurses administer acupuncture anaesthesia. They can proceed to study medicine and become doctors if they show proper clinical and political attitude.

Hospitals and Clinics

There are large hospitals in Chinese cities and smaller ones in communes. Most of them are general hospitals, but there are some special institutions, such as the Institute of Neurosurgery in Peking. The bed capacity varies anywhere from twenty to a thousand beds. The latest figure on the total number of hospitals and hospital beds is not available, but it is estimated at about 15,000 hospitals with 600,000 beds. In addition to this, there are 200,000 clinics and health stations in rural areas. The People's Liberation army has its own hospital but data on this is not available.

Since the Cultural Revolution, the hospitals do not have any administrators. They are governed by revolutionary committees composed of representatives of various categories of hospital personnel, such as doctors, nurses, technicians, and usually a Communist party member who is a non-medical man.

The large hospitals have many departments, just as any modern hospital in the Western world does. There are facilities for various surgical specialties such as chest surgery, neurosurgery, orthopedic surgery and eye surgery. Medical specialties such as cardiology and neurology are also represented and there are special wards for traditional medicine. Some hospitals have units for paraplegia or for burns.

Generally the hospitals are quite clean and well run. The laboratory service is usually adequate and modern, although in some of the smaller hospitals the equipment is old. A brief description of some of my visits to hospitals will give an insight into their function.

1. Commune Hospital in New China Commune near Canton:

This hospital has twenty beds and serves a population of 60,000 as well as controlling twenty-two clinics. It has a staff of thirty medical workers which is divided as follows:

Eight doctors
Five nurses
Three gynecologists and obstetricians
Four nerve doctors
Two public health workers
Four herbalists
Four doctors of Chinese medicine

The chief medical officer is a surgeon, Dr. Pan Chuan-Li. A graduate of a Western type of medical school, he has had post-graduate training in general surgery. He came to this hospital about five years ago in response to an appeal from Chairman Mao for doctors to go out into the countryside. All surgery except thoracic surgery and neurosurgery is done in this hospital. Usually one major operation is performed daily. There is a good laboratory for basic laboratory work and a well-stocked pharmacy. Herbs are grown in the hospital compound and drugs are manufactured in the pharmacy.

2. Huashan Hospital in Shanghai:

This 1,000 bed hospital has a staff of 720. It is a regional referral hospial, and is also affiliated with two medical schools. The hospital assigns a doctor to each patient. But the patient has the freedom to reject this choice and choose his own doctor and also whether he wants Chinese or Western treatment. Most of the patients, however, accept whatever doctor or treatment is suggested.

A large hospital like this has a portion of the staff (in this case sixty) in the countryside running mobile medical clinics. The hospital is run by a revolutionary committee, but the majority of members of this committee are medical men.

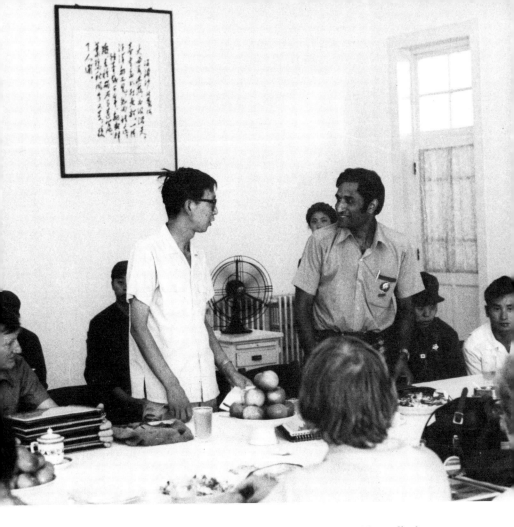

Dr. Jain confers with medical
personnel at Bethune
International Peace Hospital.

3. Medical Institute in Nanking City:

This 500 bed hospital which was founded in 1951 has a staff of 550. There are twenty departments and a special unit which treats burns with a combination of herbs and surgery. (Results of their treatment will be discussed in another chapter.) There is also a department of nuclear medicine with facilities available for liver and brain scans to detect tumors of these organs. The hospital is run by a revolutionary committee. The chief spokesman is a non-medical man. Department heads were not allowed to talk to me directly. Our conversation took place through the spokesman.

4. Bethune International Peace Hospital:

Located in Shi Jia Zhuang, this is probably the best hospital I visited. It was built as a memorial to Dr. Norman Bethune who died in service with the Chinese Army of Mao Tse-tung. Although it's run by the People's Liberation Army, twenty percent of the patients are civilians. They have 800 beds and 300 staff members out of which 60 are doctors. At any time, one-third of the staff of this hospital is on rotation duty in the countryside operating about 100 mobile clinics. They also have trained 500 barefoot doctors in the last three years.

The operating rooms are well-equipped, clean and air conditioned. There are twelve patients in each ward. Most of them had liver and gastrointestinal ailments, but were ambulatory and required a minimum of nursing care.

The overall medical care in China is not very expensive. Hospital buildings are very modest and only those people who really require hospitalization are admitted. If any patient misuses the hospital facilities or shows up too often with minor conditions, he is not admitted to the hospital. The Chinese save a lot on manpower and are able to manage with only a fraction of the nursing staff required in a modern North American hospital. The Chinese hospitals are self-sufficient. Their pharmacies are well-stocked with drugs grown in their backyard gardens. They manufacture their own vaccines, bandages, and other supplies.

Comparison of Hospital Facilities in China and North America

It is difficult to compare the North American hospital facilities with those of China. The number of beds per unit of population is not an adequate index because of the variable length of the patients' stay. There is approximately one hospital bed available for about 8,000 Chinese. In my own community in Canada, there are approximately 600 hospital beds for a population of approximately 150,000 making it one hospital bed for 250 people. However, we have a long waiting list of patients who cannot get into the hospital because of a bed shortage. In China, there are no such problems. It is difficult to comprehend this disparity. Perhaps the following points may help the reader to understand the situation:

1. In China, only very ill patients seek admission to the hospital. Most minor ailments are treated on a clinic level. In comparison, many of our hospital beds are filled with people with conditions which could have been treated outside.

2. Although no figures are available about the average hospital stay of a patient in China, from our brief observation it is much shorter than in a North American hospital. One reason for this is the very

prompt handling of new admissions. For example, a patient with a brain tumor would have the bare, minimal investigations necessary and would be operated on within four days, but in a Western hospital a patient in a similar situation might lie around for a full week undergoing all kinds of tests, sometimes for teaching purposes.

After surgery in China, the period of recovery is much shorter. One explanation for this can be found in the chapter on acupuncture anaesthesia. There are fewer post-operative complications and patients leave the hospital sometimes before they are fully recovered because they have relatives willing to take care of them. This is often not possible in North America.

Another reason for long stays in North American hospitals is lack of facilities to care for chronically-ill patients and for the very old. In China, the family unit still looks after this type of patient. There is no problem in discharging them from the hospital. In North America chronic-care patients may stay in the hospital for as long as a month just because they have no place to recuperate.

3. Many Americans with emotional disorders occupy hospital beds. Their problems vary from headaches to belly aches. A lot of expensive and extensive tests are done. When nothing is found, a patient is discharged from the hospital with the reassurance that he is healthy. All this generally takes about a week. There are very few such patients in China. Somehow or other one does not see them in hospitals. They may be screened out to various clinics.

In a private enterprise system, where a doctor is paid for services on a per visit basis, there is a tendency, on the part of some physicians, to keep a patient in the hospital longer than necessary. There are no such incentives or motivations for doctors in China. Their incomes are fixed.

The Chinese hospitals are far more simple in construction than those in North America. They look primitive in comparison to our modern American hospitals. Their furnishings are sparse and there are no luxuries. The patient sleeps on a hard, simple mattress with just a blanket to cover him. It costs the Chinese authorities less than a few dollars a day to maintain one hospital bed compared to around $70 per day in hospitals in our community. This figure is as high as $100 in some of the larger North American cities. By Western technical standards the Chinese hospitals would be very-poorly equipped, however, the Chinese have all the essential things in their hospitals and this simplicity does not detract from the treatment of the patients. Their hospitals are kept clean and their infection rate is quite low. Although the hospitals are not air-conditioned, in the hot weather patients have hand fans to cool themselves.

The Chinese save on their hospital budget by eliminating all unnecessary laboratory investigations. In our hospitals some very elaborate, expensive radiological tests are done prior to operations. The Chinese do the bare minimum and rely more on clinical judgement. This may not be an acceptable thing in a country where the facilities are available and people demand the best. A shortcut approach to medicine would create legal problems for the doctors in North America, who have to have good documentation of the patient's condition prior to surgery. Such medical legal problems do not exist in China, nor is there any mistrust of doctors by patients. The Chinese take these shortcuts purely for economic reasons. They know that their financial resources are limited and they try to make the best of what they have. In China the participation of the patient in his own care lessens the number of nursing and orderly personnel required.

In conclusion, I think that in spite of their limited economic resources the Chinese provide adequate and acceptable medical care for their population. If any comparison has to be drawn, it is not between China and the West at present, but what China was prior to Liberation and what they are now. Certainly the improvements they have made in their medical care since 1949 far outstrip the rate of progress that medicine has advanced in the Western nations. With improvements in their economic status, I feel they will tend to provide more hospital beds with more facilities and more commodities for their patients.

4

Venereal Disease and Drug Abuse Conquered

Public health in China is closely related to the social life of the people. Here is a brief account of contemporary Chinese society.

Social Life

The Chinese people are indoctrinated by Communist philosophy. Mao and his selected writings, *The Red Book,* have a stronger influence on the people than any past religion. The Chinese are very traditional people and many of their customs have remained unchanged throughout their history. One example is the family unit. Although there are large communes in the rural areas, family units are still preserved.

There are few old people in China at the present time. Most of those who would now comprise the older generation either were killed during the 1949 struggle for liberation or succumbed to one of the variety of diseases endemic to China in the past. The surviving old-timers are highly-respected in the Chinese society. They live with their children and grandchildren. During my stay I had several occasions to visit families where three generations were living in the same house.

The tradition of caring for the old at home solves many of the social and medical problems that our North American society faces. The grandpa and grandma are members of the household helping with the work and babysitting for their grandchildren. In contrast to this, the plight of the aged in North America is pathetic. Because of the longer life span in North America, there are more aged people and the problem is magnified. There are numerous elderly people lying in hospitals, institutions for the chronically-ill and homes for the aged. Those who are healthy and able to live outside on their own are generally very lonely.

The vast majority of our people do not enjoy this stage of their lives because our basic social structure breaks down the family unit. Due to unrestricted travel and un-limited opportunities for moving around, we have a large drifting population in North America. In many instances, parents live far away from their children and do not get to see them very often. This serves to widen the generation gap peculiar to our society. Under these circumstances the elderly feel alienated from the younger people who constitute the major segment of society.

The financial resources available to our senior citizens do not replace the human element. An elderly person detached from his family is rarely happy, no matter how many diversions are provided. I feel the Eastern way of treating the elderly is far superior. They are considered useful members of the society. Regardless of changes in the political philosophy, where we might anticipate a greater divergence of opinion between generations, there has been no disruption of family life. In this respect, we may indeed have something to learn from the Chinese.

Even when the Western influence tends to separate the Chinese families geographically, they try to preserve family unity. Our travel guides, male and female, mostly married, had to be away from their spouses for as long as two to three months. But they visited with them at every opportunity. This is an unusual circumstance as people usually live close to their place of work. When employment requires people to live a distance from their parents, the government provides holidays with paid transportation so those workers can visit their families at least once a year. Although this leads to some break-up of family life, it doesn't weaken family ties.

The Chinese consider children their most precious possession and lavish them with love and care. Working mothers have to leave their children at nurseries, but they visit them on work breaks. The Chinese children are not emotionally deprived and have none of the problems of the children in Western society, who are often neglected by their parents.

Although parents in North America live with their children, they seldom spend adequate time with them. In many families, when the father comes home from work the children are packed off to watch TV and then they are put to bed. They don't see their parents all day and don't see very much of them at night.

Chinese children don't watch TV alone. And they accompany their parents when they go for an evening of entertainment. It is not considered socially unacceptable to take the children. In China, children are welcome at a ballet or a theatre. I do not feel that a mother must be with her child all day long. As long as she sees the child at regular intervals and spends considerable time with him

during the evening, there is no danger of emotional depri-
vation. If a child is left at a nursery, the type of care
provided there is very important too.

The Chinese are sexually puritanical. Premarital
and extra-marital sex is not common. Sublimation of
energy in constructive work and political ideology keep
most of the Chinese from sexual adventures. There are
few opportunities for this type of activity since there are
no bars, night clubs, or prostitutes and the opportunity for
business travel is rare. This way of life is partially responsible for a low incidence of venereal disease.

Personal Habits

The Chinese are very clean, moderate people.
Although they dress modestly, their clothes are washed
frequently. Drinking water is boiled, thus getting rid of
disease producing organisms. Weak tea is preferred to
alcohol. The potent alcoholic beverages such as Mai-Tai,
are used only for toasting on special occasions. Throughout my stay in China I never saw anyone who had drunk
too much alcohol.

The Chinese do not have a drug problem such as
we have in the Western society. They eliminated this problem after the liberation. Non-medical use of drugs is unknown. Our inquiries about marihuana, LSD, and other
drugs that Americans misuse, drew empty glances from
people. Many people in Western society think that the
Chinese smoke opium but there was no evidence of this in
modern China. Opium is under strict control of three
central governments and only enough is produced for the
medical needs of the country. There is no export of opium.
The only vice, from a health standpoint, seems to be smok-

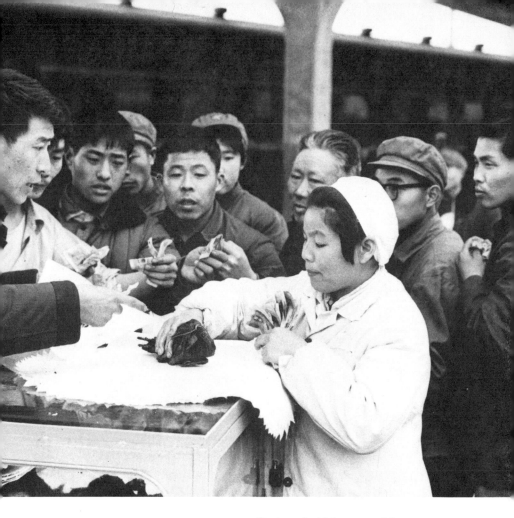

Duck and chicken, as sold to
Chinese travelers in this
railroad station, suggest a
nutritious alternative to usual
American snack foods.

ing. There are some moves to discourage people from smoking as the incidence of lung cancer is rising.

The Chinese are very honest and I did not lose a single article in China although the hotel doors are unlocked.

Nutrition

The Chinese eat well. There is plenty of inexpensive food available, and the general level of nutrition, particularly in the younger people is good. Throughout my one month stay I did not see a single case of malnutrition, either in a hospital or on the street. One of the reasons the Chinese maintain a high level of nutrition is the variety in their diet. In an average Chinese meal, there are at least five different items which vary from vegetables to meat to fish. The Chinese style of cooking does not destroy food as much as some other Eastern cooking styles do (particularly that of India). The Chinese cook their vegetables over low heat and never deep-fry them. They consume plenty of fresh fruits and use both fresh and preserved eggs. One thing which is conspicuously missing from an average Chinese meal is milk. But with the variety in their diet the lack of milk does not seem to make much difference.

The Chinese do not eat very many refined and processed foods like we do. There are no boxed cereals and very little packaged foods of any kind. They do have bottled soft drinks, however, comparable to the soft drinks we have here, but they are not consumed in large quantities. The commonest Chinese drink is still weak tea with no milk, sugar or lemon added. Since the children eat very little candy, they have relatively good teeth and less incidence of caries. But the children like chewing gum, which the Chinese have recently started to manufacture, and approach foreign visitors asking for it.

I did not feel that the Chinese had any bad eating habits. Although their food is bulky, I did not see any obesity. The basis of their diet is rice with meat, fish or vegetables added but there are some changes being made and more and more wheat products are being introduced. This is for economic rather than dietary reasons. Rice is more expensive than wheat. The Chinese sell their surplus rice to other Eastern countries in order to earn foreign exchange with which they can buy wheat, at much cheaper prices, from countries such as Canada. In addition to this, they are growing wheat, using varieties which produce maximum yield.

Mental Health

The Chinese way of life is not stressful and does not produce many neurotic or emotional disorders. However, there are some cases of mental illnesses, mostly among older people who could not cope with the stress of political changes. High officials in the Communist Party are also subject to stresses which sometimes lead to psychological or physical ailments. Stomach ulcers and heart disease have the same frequency among professional people in China as in the Western countries.

The care of the mentally ill is another blend of old and new medicine and has strong political overtones, particularly in group therapy sessions. Although sleeping pills and tranquilizers are available, without prescription, in any drug store, their consumption is merely a fraction of what is being consumed in Western countries. Shock therapy is not used in China for mental disorders and acupuncture is used only occasionally. Since acupuncture has systemic effects it is possible that it may prove effective in the future for treating mental disorders.

Emphasis on Sports

One of the reasons for the good health of the Chinese people is their mass participation in sports. Twenty years ago, Chairman Mao issued the call, "Promote culture and sports and build up the people's health."

The Chinese are famous for their competence in ping-pong, but they indulge in other sports as well. They have a special system of exercises called T'ai-Chi which is similar to Yoga but much more complicated. T'ai-Chi, an ancient system which has been modified, is usually practiced in groups.

All age groups take part in exercises. I saw dignified old men romping with their grandchildren in public parks. In one park, I saw a net stretched across the entrance gate. People were playing badminton there at six o'clock in the morning. Soccer and basketball are also favorite pastimes. Swimming is very popular and there are adequate facilities. Most communities have nice swimming pools which can be used for a nominal fee. Although the Chinese aren't known for their activity in track events, I saw some young Chinese boys practicing middle-distance running. But they did not appear to have had anyone coaching them. Bicycling, of course, is more a means of transportation than it is a sport. Most of the people use bicycles if they have to commute any distance which is outside their walking range.

Jogging is not very popular and when I went out running every day, I drew curious glances from the people.

Control of Epidemic Diseases

For centuries, China was plagued by epidemic diseases such as malaria, smallpox, cholera, tuberculosis, and schistosomiasis. Now, these diseases are practically wiped out. The Chinese have accomplished this with mass campaigns for the control of flies and mosquitoes and by cleaning the litter from their streets.

The Chinese have used DDT very extensively for eradication of flies and mosquitoes. I asked some of the physicians and public health workers if they were concerned about the toxic effects of DDT or apprehensive about it altering the life cycles in the environment. I also asked if the insects had shown any signs of developing a resistance to DDT.

My host, a public health worker, said they have not had any problem with DDT and do not anticipate any. This was the consensus. It is rather difficult to comprehend in view of what we know about the role of DDT in interfering with the environment. Perhaps the Chinese were able to eradicate these pests before they developed resistance. There was no evidence of any research to develop non-chemical methods of pest control, nor alternative chemicals to DDT.

The Chinese have a very effective immunization program, and more than 90 percent of their children have been inoculated against tuberculosis (BCG vaccination), diphtheria, whooping cough, tetanus, polio, measles, meningitis, and encephalitis.

One of the best examples of disease control is that of schistosomiasis (snail fever), which has a snail as an intermediary host. In answer to Chairman Mao's instructions "Snail fever must be wiped out," 30,000,000 people in rice growing areas of South China launched campaigns which have practically destroyed all snails.

Venereal Disease

Shanghai had the highest incidence of venereal disease in the world prior to liberation. Gangsters controlled the prostitution dens which were immediately closed after liberation. Dr. Hatem began pioneer work in the treatment of venereal disease. According to him, 80 percent of the 70,000 prostitutes in the Peking-Tiensin area were infected with venereal diseases. His clinics treated about 1,200 girls every two weeks. They were successful in rehabilitating most of the girls. Many who were cured went to work on farms, others were trained to be laboratory technicians. Since there was no stigma attached to their past many of them are now married.

These campaigns were duplicated in other cities. By 1957, all of China had been covered except Tibet. Venereal disease in China was practically eliminated. Although there is still an Institute of Venereology and Skin Diseases (it used to be in Peking but the present location is unknown) where the work on venereal diseases is being carried on, there are not enough cases to show to the medical students.

Venereal diseases have plagued the West, in an ever increasing spiral, over the last three generations. Our approach is to have venereal disease clinics which are supposed to detect and treat new cases. It has been recognized for a long time that prostitution and promiscuous sexual activity are major causes of the spread of venereal disease. But because of the basic moral structure of our society most prostitutes will not utilize the clinics' facilities and the disease goes uncontrolled.

Prostitution is difficult to control in a free Western society. Western nations which have prohibited prostitution have not been able to control venereal diseases. As a matter of fact, the incidence of venereal diseases has usually gone up. The people who control prostitution go underground and then there is no means of medically checking the prostitutes. Although there is nothing so ideal as the Chinese approach to eradication of venereal diseases, an alternative would be to legalize prostitution and have strict medical controls over it.

Population Control

The Chinese have very effective birth control programs. Propaganda billboards are everywhere, in factories, clinics, and on the streets. The barefoot doctors are engaged in a nation-wide campaign to change the thinking of the Chinese people, who traditionally have had larger families. Family planning clinics were set up in most hospitals and communes as far back as 1966 and by 1969 family planning was an important state objective.

According to Dr. Lin, a Peking gynecologist, the infant mortality in rural China was 100 per 100,000 people prior to the liberation. It has now dropped to 9 per 100,000 people. The rate of population growth in Shanghai was 40 per 1,000. It has dropped to 6-7 per 1,000. Compared to the birth rate of the United States, (17-18 per 1,000) this is remarkably low. The birth rate in rural China is still three to four times larger than in big cities, but they are making progress in curbing it. One of the factors in the drop of the birth rate is the later age at which the Chinese now marry—the rural girls delay marriage to the ages of 19-23 and the city girls until 23-25. Birth control pills and contraceptive devices are provided by the state without charge. The use of herbal drugs as contraceptives is being researched and sterilization (for both men and women), as well as abortions, are easily obtained.

All the different methods of abortion known in the West are practiced in China including D & C (dilation and curettage) as well as suction (evacuation method of abortion). They are also experimenting with the use of herbs to induce abortion as well as with acupuncture. Since acupuncture can alter the activity of the internal organs, it is reasonable to suppose that acupuncture, performed at a properly selected point, can induce uterine contractions and expel the products of conception, thus resulting in abortion without the hazard of a surgical procedure.

Maternal Welfare

During pregnancy women visit hospital clinics, regularly, on an outpatient basis. Medical workers, closely supervised by physicians, are responsible for both prenatal and postnatal care. Generous maternity leave (eight weeks) with pay and other benefits is given. Most of the deliveries are done at home by midwives. But the complicated deliveries are done in a hospital.

Child Care

There are three programs for child care in China:
1. From age 56 days, when the mother's maternity leave ends, until one-and-one-half years the child can be left in a nursing room at the mother's place of employment. Here a mother may go and breast-feed her child.
2. Nurseries are run for children from age one-and-one-half to three years. If grandparents don't take care of a child, he enters a nursery. Some of these nurseries are open twenty-four hours a day to accommodate children whose parents work at night.
3. Kindergartens are attended by children age three to seven, then the child enters primary school. China's kindergartens are very interesting institu-

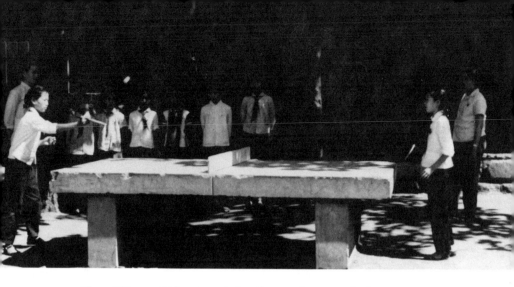

These Chinese children are playing the popular game of ping-pong.

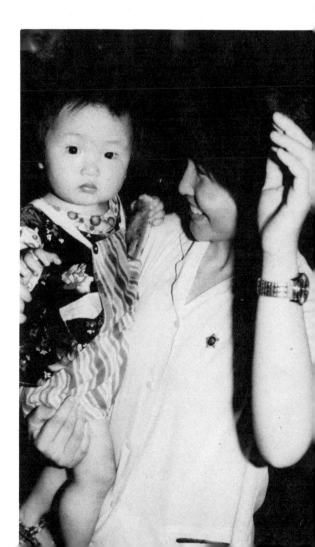

Obviously, Chinese
children are well-cared
for and much loved.

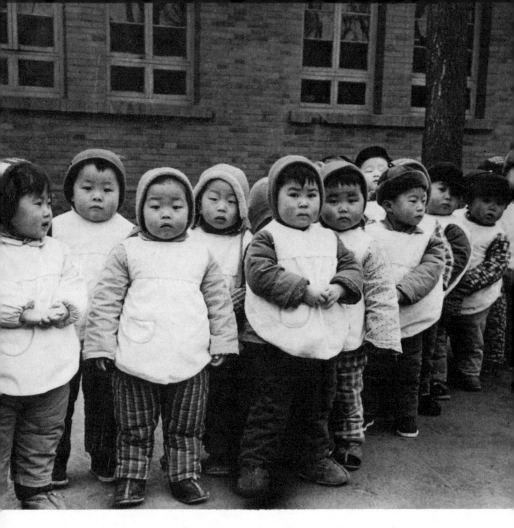

These Chinese kindergarten
children wear layers of clothing
to protect them against the
cold of the Northern Provinces.

tions. Basic education is started at this age and it is the time when philosophical and cultural values are implanted. This is the children's first experience in communal living. They learn Mao's articles pertaining to the love of work as peasants and soldiers. They are also taught to love physical labor and to sacrifice themselves in order to serve the people and help the revolution. The atmosphere in a kindergarten is revolutionary, even to the posters on the walls.

Children participate in many sports, including ping-pong. They have cultural activities in the form of plays, singing, and music, all of which again are revolutionary in theme. As mentioned earlier, the children are well-cared for and are not deprived of their parents' love. Most of the kindergartens are day institutions and the children go home and spend the evenings with their families. Kindergarten children are very well behaved. When I asked a teacher in a kindergarten how the Chinese handle problem children, she said they do not punish them, but just talk things over with them and this usually solves the problem.

The Chinese people have made great strides in the field of Public Health and at present are one of the healthiest nations in the East. Elimination of major diseases, which plague other Eastern nations, was achieved only by a mass effort guided by Mao Tse-tung's philosophy, which states in one lesson *(The Foolish Old Man Who Removed the Mountain)* that nothing is impossible. The Chinese people have proven this.

5

A Different Attitude toward Medical Education

Medical Education

As the medical schools were closed during the Cultural Revolution, the exact number functioning today is not known. They have just started to re-open these schools during the last two years.

The most drastic change in the curriculum has been the reduction in the length of study from six to three years. However, there is still no uniform medical curriculum. Medical schools have attempted to eliminate irrelevant subjects. The following quotation from an article in *China's Medicine* in 1968 gives an idea of this attitude. "The curriculum required students to study as long as six or even eight years. But after graduation they were unable to treat independently even the most frequently encountered diseases. Leaving the big hospital with its laboratory and modern equipment they found themselves at their wit's end. In the course of six years 3/4 of their time was spent studying textbooks and reciting abstract theories. The preclinical subjects differed so sharply from the clinical work that the student could find no effective use for the supposedly basic theories which had been drilled into them. The education in the medical colleges over the years was carried out after the fashion of the stuffing and fattening of a Peking duck. The students memorized the subjects for the examination and once their ordeals were over, all was well and forgotten." They now use the precepts of Chairman Mao's three in one principle.

1. The student can teach the teacher.
2. The teacher teaches the student.
3. The student teaches the student.

Selection of Students

Admission to medical school is open to soldiers, workers, and peasants. There is no direct admission from high school to a university or medical school. Among the criteria for selection:

1. The individual's degree of motivation to study medicine is considered.

2. The applicant is evaluated by his commune as to whether he is a good worker and a bona fide proletarian, who identifies with the masses.

3. He also needs a recommendation by the Communist Party stating that he has studied Mao Tsetung's teachings.

4. He has to be accepted by the Revolutionary Committee of the medical school.

Students usually start medical school when they are between seventeen and twenty years of age. Many of these students are already barefoot doctors or trained nurses.

A Typical Chinese Medical School Curriculum.. .. ..

> *9 months*—In medical school. Study of basic subjects such as anatomy, physiology, microbiology, biochemistry, and traditional Chinese medicine
>
> *3 months*—Military training. Physical fitness and manual labor—this period is usually spent in the country
>
> *6 months*—Lectures on clinical subjects such as medicine, surgery and obstetrics in teaching hospitals
>
> *3 months*—Manual labor, military training and physical fitness
>
> *9 months*—Practical medical work in the country —supervised by teachers. Part of this training is studying herbs, their uses, the study and practice of acupuncture, and the study of public health
>
> *3 months*—At the university hospital studying clinical work
>
> *3 months*—Vacation, military training, and physical fitness
>
> *Total*   Three years.

As one might notice, there is a stress on physical fitness. This is because medicine is considered a "strenuous profession".

Medical School Curricula in North America

There is no uniform policy of medical education in North America, although most of the medical schools have a four year program. Prior to entrance to medical school, students are required to have four years of college education. Some of the medical students have an even higher education. A few have Ph.D's in other scientific subjects.

There has been considerable re-assessment of the curriculum in the North American medical schools which in some schools has resulted in reducing the period of study from four to three years and substituting internship in the fourth year. However, the basic difference remains in the curriculum itself. Most of the medical schools still have too many lectures and academic studies on basic subjects which may not have much practical value. Whether placing less importance on basic academic subjects will impair the quality of a physician is still being debated. A physician is faced with an increasing amount of reading material which embraces investigations of other physicians, as well as new discoveries. In spite of this, a medical student today has less studying than his counterpart of a decade ago. This is due to the exclusion of some of the more redundant material from the medical curriculum.

The other basic difference is in the premedical education. In North America, we feel that a doctor should be a well-educated man first and a doctor second. This is the reason for requiring four years of college to prepare a student for medical school. In China, such an education prior to going into medicine would be superfluous and wasteful. There is no doubt in my mind that a student who has a good academic education will become a better doctor, but this is not a practical proposition in every country, particularly those with limited resources. The

Chinese medical curriculum is tailored to meet their needs. In China, a physician's political knowledge and service to the people is valued far more than his knowledge of fine arts. The North American medical curriculum produces physicians who are better suited to deal with the North American public. It is impossible to make a fair comparison.

In China, due to elimination of scholastic examinations the question of measuring academic excellence does not arise. They do not create homogenious categories of students based on their marks—a system which does not appear to be very practical even in our Western society which is accustomed to set standards and examinations.

It is unfortunate that most nurses in North America who would like to become physicians have to go back to college before they can enter medical school. This eliminates many potentially good physicians. In China, a well-motivated medical worker can start medical school without much of an educational background.

The following story, "I Will Study To Become a Good Doctor" by Hsu Yun-hsin, a student at Peking Medical College, is interesting and is reprinted from the *Peking Medical Review* (May 12, 1972):

I was a barefoot doctor in my village before I went to college.

"I had taken a short hospital training course to start with, and then got clinical experience and learned the use of various folk prescriptions as I went along.

"Acupuncture was in great demand at my people's commune. So I studied it, learning from experienced acupuncture doctors, and applying the acupuncture needles on various points of my body to obtain experience. Through such repeated practice, I came to know thoroughly several dozen points on the human body and experienced the sensations of numbness, swelling, aching, and pain at each point.

"A patient with stomach ulcers came in one night. He was having spasms of excruciating pain. I gave him several different drugs, but all to no avail. He then asked me if I could do acupuncture. I told him that up to now I had only used it on myself. He asked me to try it on him. I inserted needles at three different points in his body which could cure ulcers. After I had made two insertions, he felt the pain diminishing, and when I had left the needles in the different positions for twenty more minutes, he declared it had completely stopped. This initial success gave me great encouragement.

"High blood pressure had plagued 68-year-old Uncle Chen of my village for years. In 1969, he became partially paralyzed. No amount of medicine worked. He could not go often to the commune hospital because of his conditions, so the hospital sent a doctor to teach me how to give him acupuncture treatment. I went regularly to Uncle Chen's, using the new acupuncture treatment method on him as well as needling the ear. The old man got better. A month later, he recovered. I was indescribably happy to have been able to ease the suffering of poor and lower-middle peasants like him.

"Though I had then mastered acupuncture and knew the use of some of the simpler drugs, both Chinese and Western, and had cured some common diseases in the countryside with them, I was unable to deal with more complicated cases. I could only give such patients preliminary aid and recommend that they go to the hospital. I often thought at the time of how nice it would be if I could study to improve my medical skill and heal more patients.

"My wish came true in winter 1970. I was recommended to study at Peking Medical College, and became one of its first students from worker, peasant or soldier origin.

"I will never forget the night before I left for college. My home was full of people. Many poor and lower-middle peasants had come to see me off. Old Chang remarked: 'What wonderful times I have lived to see, when our children are going to college!' Another old man, Hsu, added: 'There were so many epidemics in the old days . . . How many children used to die in spring and summer! . . .' One grandmother, Li said: 'Remember 1934? Cholera must have killed dozens of people in the village that time . . .'

"So the 'send-off' became a meeting in which the evils of the old society were condemned, and the good things of the new praised. It was late in the night when the gathering broke up.

"Whenever my studies give me difficulties now that I'm in college, I recall that night. The accusation against the old society and the hopes the village folk placed in me always give me new strength. I've finished the basic required courses, and am now taking clinical courses at one of the college hospitals.

"Like the people back home, I too am looking forward to the day when I will go back a competent doctor, to heal sickness and pain among my people."

On graduation the students return to the communes from which they came, thus solving the problem of placement. There are no examinations during or after the training program. There are no grades and no competition between students. The only reason a student may fail to graduate is because of ill health, and in this situation he can return to study when his health improves. There is no tuition fee and the students are paid a modest stipend to pay their expenses while they live in a residence on the campus of the medical school. After graduation, the new doctors are expected to keep interested in recent developments by constant study and self-criticism. They also study Western medicine by reading our medical journals.

Postgraduate Education

There are no set programs for postgraduate education. To train as a specialist, a Chinese doctor spends two or three years working under established specialists in a big teaching hospital. If he is considered competent, he is allowed to restrict his practice to his specialty. Again there are no qualifying examinations. The training of specialists is limited to the need for them, so no surplus of doctors is produced in any field of medicine.

In comparison, North American postgraduate education is very elaborate. The residency training system, which has evolved during the past fifty years, involves training an M.D. for four to five years, in a teaching hospital setting, to prepare him to become a specialist. This training is programmed to give a resident increasingly more responsibility. He is exposed to many disciplines of medicine related to his specialty. At the end of the training period, there are examinations which a candidate must pass before he becomes a fully-qualified specialist.

In Canada it is almost essential for a doctor to have a degree in his specialty before he can practice it or get an appointment to a hospital. This is an excellent system, but it has its drawbacks. No two candidates require the same amount of training time to become good specialists; there are some specialists who are unable to pass the examination, who would be competent to practice their specialty; there is no control over the number of specialists produced.

The number of positions available for postgraduate students or residents is small in certain fields and abundant in others. Therefore, we end up with an over-abundance of specialists in some fields and a shortage in others. For example, in psychiatry and pathology in North America most of the residency positions remain unfilled due to lack of interest. Overall, we have a higher percentage of specialists than the Chinese. In my own community 50 percent of the doctors have a specialty of one sort or another.

Although the Chinese training is more flexible, and a brilliant man, who learns fast, may become a specialist in a shorter time than a slow learner, I doubt the wisdom of abolishing examinations for postgraduate students.

Medical Training in P. L. A.

The People's Liberation Army (P.L.A.) maintains its own hospitals. They do not have a definite medical curriculum. When they need an extra doctor, they put one of their soldiers into medical training and in one to three years he is capable of carrying out general medical duties. The requirements for specialization are also flexible. Neurasthenia or nervous exhaustion appears frequently in Chinese soldiers so doctors in the P.L.A. often specialize just in this narrow field of need.

Research

Research and medical publications were suspended during the Cultural Revolution, with the exception of a few important projects. The emphasis during this period was on the practice of medicine, and only clinical research was carried out. Most of the research these days is concerned with acupuncture. It includes acupuncture anaesthesia and the use of acupuncture in the treatment of various conditions. The Chinese are also very interested in research in cancer, in the cure of paralysis, and treatment of deafness.

In comparison with the United States, China is very primitive in its research activities. Medicine is a constantly evolving science and research appears to be essential to keep it up-to-date. But it is expensive and the Chinese can ill afford it. What research China has done is significant. They have provided a theme for the research of American physicians as evidenced by the number of doctors who are investigating acupuncture and Chinese herbs.

6

The Ancient Art of Acupuncture

The most talked about facet of Chinese medicine today is acupuncture. It has become a household word and the subject of many newspaper and magazine articles within the last year. Acupuncture is not new. It has been used in China for 3,000 years and in Europe for a century. There are an estimated 2,000 practitioners of this art outside the Orient. About 700 of them are in France where there is an Institute of Acupuncture. There is some research being done by the Russians through the Soviet Academy of Sciences. During my recent visit to U.S.S.R., I tried to get some more information about this, but the Russian physicians were reluctant to talk about China and acupuncture. There are some scattered practitioners of the art in North America including one in Vancouver. About thirty practicing acupuncturists in England are attracting 10,000 British patients each week. Fifteen years ago there was only one acupuncturist in London and almost no patients. In Japan, where acupuncture is very popular, there are approximately 25,000 practitioners of this art.

It seems odd that with acupuncture being practiced in so many countries outside of China, no notice was taken of it by the medical profession in North America. The Western physicians were highly skeptical of this mysterious Eastern practice, but with the increase in publicity given to China, acupuncture gained prominence. The extensive newspaper coverage brought patients to their physicians' offices asking questions about acupuncture. North America's doctors are now interested but the lack of scientific documentation still keeps them from accepting it as an efficient method of treatment. So far neither the Chinese nor any of the European physicians who have been practicing acupuncture have been able to conclusively prove its value.

Acupuncture, as the derivation of the word implies (acus - needle; puncta - puncture), is the insertion of a needle into the skin of the human body. This is done at certain specified points to depths varying from a few millimeters to sometimes a few centimeters. These points are located on the twelve major meridians on the body each corresponding to a major organ system of the body. There are approximately 1,000 such points which have been determined by trial and error.

The Technique of Acupuncture

The very fine needles used in acupuncture are made of stainless steel. Each organ of the body is represented on the skin at a distance from the organ and is located on a particular meridian. A practitioner of acupuncture may use a chart or a mannikin to help him select

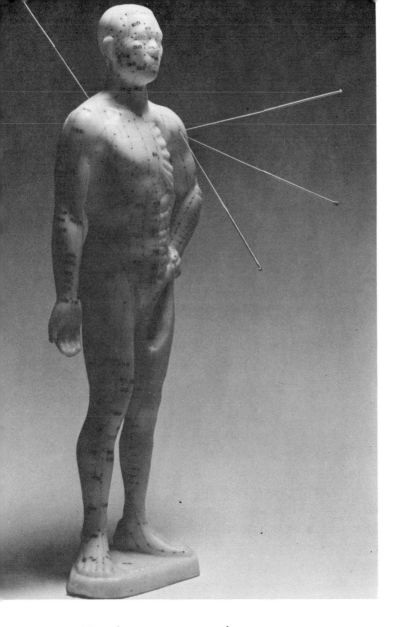

The meridians for acupuncture are shown on
this statue, which is used as a teaching aid.
Several needles have been inserted to
demonstrate the procedure.

the proper point for treatment. Some of the common points are:

1. The acupuncture point for the right lower quadrant of the abdomen is located on the outer aspect of the right knee.

2. The acupuncture point for the head is on the big toe.

3. The acupuncture point for the heart is the wrist, at the base of the little finger.

These points can also be located by measuring the skin's electrical resistance which changes at the acupuncture points.

A detailed description of the technique is beyond the scope of this work. But the following will give you a general idea of how acupuncture functions.

The needles are sterilized and inserted gently at the acupuncture point and then gradually moved with the hand. The direction of insertion of the needle, the type of movement and duration which the needle is kept in, all vary according to the patient's condition and are decided before the procedure is started. Acupuncturists avoid hitting any blood vessels, nerves, or other important organs of the body. Relief of symptoms is usually quite prompt, but sometimes the needles have to be left in for a longer period than was originally decided on. The treatments are often repeated at intervals of days, weeks or months. Recently, acupuncture needles have been made hollow thus allowing them to be used for injection of drugs through acupuncture.

Another recent innovation is the use of computers in acupuncture. Computerized mannikins are available with buttons for the symptoms. After the practitioner punches a combination of symptoms and the location of the organ, the computer lights up indicating the point where the needle should be inserted.

The Chinese have traditionally selected acupuncture points by the involved method of pulse diagnosis, which will be discussed in another chapter. The Japanese, who adopted acupuncture from the Chinese, do not use pulse diagnosis as it requires many years of experience to become proficient at it. It is impossible for a beginning practitioner to locate the acupuncture point with any degree of accuracy by this method.

The Japanese, with their flair for technology, use electronic gadgets to locate acupuncture points. Their findings are based on the alteration of skin resistance to electric current. As soon as a probe is passed over the acupuncture point, there are alterations indicated on the meters. Where there is dysfunction of the body, there will be more fluctuation at the corresponding acupuncture point.

The points selected for acupuncture are treated by insertion of needles which are stimulated electrically rather than manually. It is surprising that the acupuncture points selected this way correspond very closely to the Chinese acupuncture points. Most Western patients would be more impressed by the gadgetry of the Japanese acupuncture treatment than the simple needle insertion of the Chinese.

Theories of Acupuncture

How does a simple needle insertion relieve a patient's symptoms and cure his illness? There is as yet no scientific proof of the mode of action, only theories which I will summarize:

1. The ancient Chinese hypothesized that diseases

are due to imbalance of Yin (negative) and Yang (positive). Acupuncture restores this balance. As mentioned in Chapter I, the Chinese concept of the Universe is based on Yin and Yang. The Chinese attempt to explain this balance in terms of what we know as the autonomic or "self-governing" nervous system.

The autonomic nervous system is formed by two sets of nerves called the sympathetic and the parasympathetic. The impulses originating from these sets of nerves must always be in balance to co-ordinate organ functions and to keep the body in good health. If the sympathetic system (Yang) is stimulated, the heart beats stronger and faster, the blood pressure rises and the muscular movements of the intestine are impeded. If the parasympathetic system (Yin) is stimulated the opposite happens, that is, the heart slows down, the blood pressure falls and there is increased movement of the intestine.

There is a free association between the two components of the autonomic nervous system: the brain, and the voluntary nervous system (the part of the nervous system controlling the movements of the muscles and joints). It is accepted in the Western way of thinking that the physiological or pathological conditions in one organ of the body may influence other organs through reflex actions. For example, heat is applied to a certain part of the skin to influence internal organs connected to that area of the skin through the nervous system. Thus, there appears to be no great fundamental difference between the Western and the ancient Chinese concept of the interplay of the nervous system with the organs of the body.

The ancient Chinese belief is that the Yin and Yang energies circulate in the inner and outer parts of the body without ceasing and that within the twelve meridians the origin of an illness can be found by locating an excess or deficiency of energy. Once the site of disturbance of the energy flow is located the proper flow can be reestablished to maintain the equilibrium between Yin and Yang. In the light of Western knowledge of development of the human embryo this is not difficult to believe. We know that the skin and the nerves evolve from the same type of cells. It is highly-possible that some connection persists between the skin and the nerve which developed from the same embryonic group of cells.

2. Those that espouse the neural theory believe that the acupuncture points correspond to areas of referred pain. According to Henry Head (an English neurologist), skin pain in diseases of internal organs is located in the areas where the nerves carrying sensations enter the spinal cord at the same place as nerves supplying the corresponding internal organs. For example, left arm pain is referred from a heart disease. According to this theory, insertion of a needle into such a zone of skin stimulates the flow of impulses which alters the central nervous system function of the spinal segment involved. It either inhibits or adjusts the function of the central nervous system (particularly the autonomic nervous system, and the balance between the sympathetic and the parasympathetic components).

In 1959 Russian workers submitted some evidence to support this theory. In laboratory tests of patients with peptic ulcers, it was found that, after acupuncture, the blood content of histamine and epinephrine (which is usually elevated) returned to normal. It is possible that this adjusting effect may be mediated at a higher level than the spinal cord, for example in the thalamus (situated in the deeper part of the brain).

This theory explains why acupuncture is most effective in treatment of functional disorders of the internal organs.

3. The Gate Control Theory of Professor Melzak of McGill University can be applied to explain the effect of acupuncture and relief of pain. According to Dr. Chang Hsian-tung, Director of Acupuncture Research at Shanghai's Physiological Institute. This is somewhat similar to the theory outlined in No. 2. Nerve impulses starting from the point of needling, and those arising from the diseased organs, are conducted to the same segment of the spinal cord. The impulses from the point of acupuncture may inhibit the other impulses, thus causing relief of pain.

4. The Kim Bong Ducts theory was named after a professor of physiology in North Korea. According to him, acupuncture acts through body systems such as the circulatory system or the nervous system. He used radioactive tracers to establish the existence of a new type of conducting channel in the subepidermal layer of the skin corresponding to the classical meridians. The Chinese authorities do not agree with this.

5. The Electrical Resistance Theory exists because acupuncture points have different electrical resistance from the surrounding skin. This has been proven with electronic instruments at Lomanosov University in Moscow. The acupuncture points are located in connective tissues. This theory is

significant in explaining the alterations in the body which result from inserting needles at these points. Acupuncture points located by measuring the electrical resistance of the skin correspond closely to the classical acupuncture points. Some new points have been discovered by this technique.

6. The theory that post-hypnotic suggestion is responsible for the effectiveness of acupuncture can be dismissed on the following grounds:

   (a) There is a measurable change in the human body after acupuncture. For example, on insertion of a needle, there is peristaltic movement of the intestine which can be observed under an x-ray fluoroscope.
   (b) Acupuncture is effective in children and animals although they are not good subjects for, hypnosis.
   (c) Acupuncture needles at the wrong points of the body can lead to aggravation of symptoms.
   (d) The treatment has been used on millions of people throughout China over the past several years. It is difficult to believe that this vast number of people were all hypnotized.

7. Recent work has been done by the Soviet Union using high-voltage and high-frequency electrical fields and photographs to display a small flare emitting from the skin. They claim that the flares are plasmic and some of them correspond to acupuncture points. Further work on this theory is being done in the Soviet Union.

Research in Acupuncture

The basic research in acupuncture being done by the Chinese at the Institute of Physiology in Shanghai was not interrupted during the Cultural Revolution. Dr. Hsian-Tung, the Chinese scientist in charge of this project, studied anatomy and physiology of the nervous system at Yale University (1936-37) and Rockefeller Institute (1949-54). His team of sixteen researchers conducts three types of experiments on dogs.

1. The first set of experiments is designed to determine the role of the hypothalamus (part of the brain controlling the autonomic nervous system) in acupuncture.

2. In the second set, impulses from the area of skin going to a certain segment of the spinal cord, and impulses going from that segment to various parts of the body, are monitored and measured precisely.

3. In the third set of experiments, a cut is made in the skin. The pain impulses are recorded, acupuncture is done and the pain impulses are recorded again. This demonstrates the blocking of the impulses at a more peripheral level.

These experiments are being done objectively and the results (yet unpublished) will be very significant.

Diseases in Which Acupuncture Has Proven To Be Useful

1. *Nervous System:* Tension headaches, migraine, neuralgias, sciatica, tics, and fainting spells.

2. *Digestive System:*   Enteritis, gastric ulcers, dyspepsia, constipation, diarrhea, liver dysfunction and gallbladder disease. It is claimed that gallstones have been passed under acupuncture treatment.

3. *Cardiovascular:*   Angina, palpitations, high blood pressure.

4. *Genito-Urinary System:*   Some types of renal colic, bladder spasm, dysmenorrhea, menopausal symptoms, impotence, and frigidity. Cases have been described where renal stones have passed and pain was relieved with acupuncture treatment alone.

5. *Skin:*   Dermatitis, acne, eczema.

6. *Psychiatric Disturbances:*   Neurasthenia, fatigue, and insomnia.

7. *Respiratory Ailments:*   Asthma, bronchitis, recurrent colds, and pulmonary congestion.

8. *Miscellaneous Conditions:*   Backache due to a variety of causes. There is dramatic relief of muscle spasms on insertion of acupuncture needles. Backache due to tumor and disc disease does not respond well.

Diseases in Which Acupuncture Is Useless:

1. Paralysis resulting from stroke or head injury.

2. Cardiac Arrhythmias: according to Dr. Fan Chi (a Peking cardioligist who is involved in a research

project in the treatments of cardiac arrhythmia) there has not been any proof that acupuncture can control the disturbances of the cardiac rhythm. He still relies on established Western drugs for these conditions.

In general, those diseases where there is disturbance of physiological function respond permanently to acupuncture, but where there is anatomical abnormality, acupuncture can only relieve the symptoms temporarily.

Brief Description of Personal Observation on Acupuncture Treatment

1. A fifty-year old Chinese male was seen in a factory clinic. While lifting a heavy weight, he had suffered an acute sprain of the back and was not able to straighten up. He came to the clinic bent over and complaining of severe back pain. After a quick examination by the clinic doctor, four acupuncture needles were inserted in his back. They were left in for a period of ten minutes while the patient lay on his stomach. When the needles were removed, the patient was able to get up from the examining table, stand upright, walk out of the clinic free from pain, and go back to work. This was the most dramatic demonstration of the value of acupuncture in relieving acute muscular pain that I witnessed.

2. The second patient, seen in the same factory clinic, had developed pain in the right wrist while working. After a doctor had examined his wrist and found no evidence of disease (no x-rays were taken) acupuncture needles were inserted at acupuncture points around the right ear. After a

period of half an hour the patient had not received any relief from the pain in his wrist. Then the doctors planned to x-ray the wrist to find out what was wrong. The Western medical approach to a problem like this is immediate diagnostic x-rays. This eliminates the danger, present in the Chinese treatment, of letting a serious condition worsen by relieving pain and thus masking symptoms.

3. A thirty-five year old Canadian sinologist traveling with us was suffering from diarrhea. He had cramps and pain on the right side of his lower abdomen. Initially he was treated with Western medications which were a combination of anti-diarrheal agents and antibiotics. He improved, but his symptoms recurred. At this stage, a Chinese acupuncturist was called to the Canadian's hotel room. The acupuncturist inserted one needle on the outer aspect of the right knee and within fifteen minutes the cramps stopped. The patient remained free from diarrhea for the next two days. Treatment had to be repeated but there was no recurrence of diarrhea during the following week. This treatment shows that acupuncture can affect the intestinal motility and relieve pain.

4. A thirty-two year old Chinese housewife came to a clinic for treatment of severe, recurring headaches. These headaches occurred almost every day and in between severe attacks she had persisting dull pain, mostly in the back of the head. There was no history of migraine headaches and her headaches did not follow a definite pattern. After a brief examination by the doctor did not reveal any sign of an intracranial condition such as tumor or hemorrhage, it was decided to use acupuncture instead of medication. The acupuncture needle was inserted over a point on her left big toe and

stimulation was given for ten minutes. The patient experienced relief of pain, but the headache recurred almost immediately. Treatment was repeated with the needle left in for a longer period. This time the patient's headache disappeared and had not returned later when she left the clinic. The doctor told her to return to him if her headaches should come back.

I was told by the attending doctor that they would make further investigations if the headaches recurred, looking for some underlying pathology in the brain. This approach seems reasonable and practical to me. The doctor did not make any diagnosis of the cause, but the cause of headaches is difficult to diagnose in Western medicine too.

I saw numerous examples of the use of acupuncture to relieve pain in the post-operative period. Instead of giving the patient a strong analgesic medication, an acupuncture needle is inserted. The *New York Times* reporter, James Reston, is one of many who has had post-operative acupuncture. It was administered successfully after he underwent an appendectomy in a hospital in Peking.

My Personal Opinion About Acupuncture

In my opinion, acupuncture definitely is effective and does have a place in the practice of medicine. However, one should be a little hesitant about accepting all the claims. Acupuncture is not a panacea. The danger of overlooking a serious illness remains a real possibility. For this reason alone, an uncontrolled practice of acupuncture in Western society would be dangerous. Modern medicine prides itself on early detection of disease and treatment before development of complications. Treating painful syndromes with acupuncture might mask symptoms and delay vital treatment, particularly if the acupuncture is done by someone who is not fully qualified in the field of medicine.

In China, acupuncturists work very closely with the medical profession. So a serious condition is seldom overlooked. The danger in North America is the development of a situation where an acupuncturist sets up an independent practice like naturopaths or chiropractors. Then a patient seeking acupuncture treatment may not have the supervision of his family physician. For example, a patient with chronic headache due to a brain tumor does not have many physical signs in the earlier stages. If he goes to an acupuncturist for relief of headaches and the headaches are temporarily relieved but keep recurring, the acupuncture treatment may be covering up symptoms of a brain tumor. An acupuncturist, who is not trained in medicine, won't recognize those recurrences as trouble signs and refer the patient to an appropriate specialist for further investigations and treatment.

In order to minimize the danger, it is imperative that acupuncture be investigated and studied by the established medical profession in North America before it becomes common practice here. The practitioners of this art should work under the supervision of, and in close collaboration with, the medical profession. The family physician must have some basic understanding of acupuncture to be able to decide which patients could benefit from it and refer them to an acupuncturist in the same way as he refers patients to a physiotherapist. If the patient does not get relief, he returns to the family physician for further tests or referral to a specialist. Another way acupuncture could become part of our medical system would be for the family physicians to study it and become acupuncturists. Certainly a scientifically trained person who studies acupuncture can practice it better and more safely than a layman.

Acupuncture is usually helpful when routine medical investigations fail to uncover the cause of pain. If the cause has been found, and cured by standard medical procedures, it does not seem reasonable to persist in using acupuncture except to relieve pain. There are many conditions, such as tumors, which acupuncture will not cure.

Role of Acupuncture in Preventive Medicine

Some acupuncturists claim they can detect an imbalance in different organs of the body by the use of acupuncture electronic needles prior to the time the patient develops the disease. This has not yet been proven scientifically but it seems valid and it plays an important role in prevention of diseases. The patient can have a "toning up" of the abnormal acupuncture points. This can roughly be equated to tuning up a car engine. One seventy-two year old acupuncturist that I know claims he has been able to maintain good health by "toning up" his acupuncture points regularly whenever there is a deficiency at one point.

7

The Role of Acupuncture in Neurological Diseases

Neurology, the branch of medicine dealing with disorders of the nervous system, has been an important part of Chinese medicine. Disorders of the nervous system constitute one of the world's most common health problems. Acupuncture is used, with varying degrees of success, to treat these disorders.

Minor Disorders of the Nervous System

1. *Headaches:* Headache is one of the most common neurological complaints seen by physicians. It can be a minor condition, or it can be a symptom of a serious disease. There are many types of headaches. The two most common types, which are treated in the doctor's office, are tension headaches and migraines. The cause and cure of migraine remains a mystery. However, in the Western system of medicine, there are drugs that will abort or

control an attack of migraine. Now research is under way to find compounds that will counteract the physiological changes which occur in the body during migraine headaches. Some of these changes are well understood by physicians, but others are not clear.

The Chinese treat migraine headache with acupuncture as well as herbal medication. But acupuncture provides only temporary relief. There is no documented, permanent cure of any patient with migraine. However, some patients who do not respond to drug treatment or do not tolerate drugs well experience relief of pain when acupuncture is used during an acute attack of migraine.

Tension headaches respond to a variety of approaches including psychotherapy and tranquilizers. This complaint occurs infrequently among the Chinese and they don't have any special treatment for it, but acupuncture is sometimes used to relax the patient and temporarily relieve the headache. Its effectiveness in alleviating a condition like tension is very difficult to assess. There is an element of suggestion involved and, since tension headaches sometimes respond to very simple treatments such as rubbing the neck, they can hardly be considered valid for evaluating a form of treatment.

2. *Dizziness:*   This is fairly frequent and is seldom an indication of any other disease in the body. Acupuncture is used to treat dizziness with varying degrees of success. As with the treatment of headaches, it is very difficult to evaluate. However, it is preferable to using drugs to suppress dizziness.

3. *Painful conditions in different parts of the body due to affliction of the peripheral nerves:*   There are many conditions, such as neuralgia of the face

or limbs due to involvement of the nerves, which may be specific or nonspecific. Sometimes these painful conditions persist even when the cause is known and is being treated. Complicated neurosurgical procedures are sometimes required to relieve pain. Acupuncture has proven very helpful in treating these painful conditions although the relief of pain is not always permanent. Further research should be done in the role of acupuncture in this area.

4. *Neurasthenia or nervous exhaustion:* This condition occurs in people who are under some strain, particularly soldiers. Reference is made previously to an interview with Dr. Kuo Shu-su. He is an army neuropsychiatrist who specializes in treating this disorder. His technique, which involves stimulation and excitation during the daytime and relaxation at night, has been largely successful. A modification of acupuncture, his method involves needles which are inserted in the occipital region (back of head) under the skin. These needles are stimulated electrically.

Treatment of the Deaf and the Mute

I was taken to Peking No. 3 Municipal School for the Deaf and Dumb. This school had 228 students and 48 teachers. We spent the whole day with them, evaluating their training techniques and the results. The school, situated in one of the suburbs of Peking, draws students mostly from the surrounding areas. They usually come from peasant families. In this residential school, the youngest student was eight years old, the oldest about twenty-three.

As an introduction, I was told that there were no facilities for training people with this kind of disability prior to the Cultural Revolution. In old China, it was customary to teach certain trades to people with these handicaps. They spent their lives at menial tasks, such as weaving. This information was given to me by one of the students who had been unable to speak when she entered the school. She sang a song for us, which translated into English goes as follows:

"Withered for a thousand years the wisteria puts forth new sprouts,
After ten thousand years the iron tree bursts into flower.
Thanks to our great leader Chairman Mao,
Deaf-mutes today regain their speaking power."

The student was a sixteen year old girl who had come to the school at age two quite deaf and dumb.

We were told that treatment of the deaf and dumb is done with acupuncture and evolved in 1968 as an effort of the People's Liberation Army medical workers. A lot of investigations and experimentation went into the development of the treatment and most of these experiments were done by the Army medical workers on their own bodies. We saw a demonstration given by an army doctor who put needles into his body. Some of the points which he selected to put needles are forbidden zones in the ancient treatise on acupuncture.

After this brief introduction, we were taken around to see the actual training and progress in the classes. Then we saw acupuncture treatment being given. This latter was not a pleasant experience as the youngsters did not look forward to daily needle treatments. They sat in ordinary classrooms and the army medical workers went from one seat to another sticking needles into their arms and ears. Although no child cried (I never saw a Chinese child cry), they did indicate their dislike for this procedure by grimacing. What impressed me more than the acupuncture treatments were the speech therapy classes. Both teachers and students work very hard using political, ideological themes for practicing voice.

In the discussion that followed our visit to the school, emphasis was placed on developing a new acupuncture point for treatment of the deaf and dumb. The medical workers are particularly anxious to locate points which will stimulate speech. They said that the ancient Chinese compendium on acupuncture and moxibustion mentioned Ya Men points (under the chin), but it was forbidden to put the needles deeply into these points. The medical workers at the school insert the needles deeper than what is considered a safe limit. But they first experimented on themselves. When they tried this on the children they found that it was quite effective in stimulating speech. According to their figures, they have a success rate of about 30 percent over a period of one year of treating deaf and dumb children. Once deafness has been overcome, further acupuncture treatments produce the return of speech in 70 percent of those children. Ten percent of the children were resistant to acupuncture treatment.

I asked the medical workers about the causes of the children's deafness, but I got no specific answers. They merely listed general causes of deafness which occur anywhere, such as infection of the brain, injuries to the hearing nerve and other congenital disorders. They claim that they have kept audiographic records of patients' hearing, but no such records were available for my examination.

I find it very difficult to evaluate the effectiveness of this form of acupuncture therapy. Part of the improvement is certainly due to the good speech therapy given these children, who previously had no treatment at all.

Children in the Peking school appeared to be happy. They are discharged from the school when they regain their hearing and speech, and the acupuncture treatments are stopped when a child can hear at a distance of two meters.

Treatment on Infantile Polio

Poliomyelitis is a disease of the nervous system in which portions of the spinal cord are afflicted with a virus that causes paralysis of the extremities. This is considered an irreversable process. However, there are many examples of people who have suffered from polio as children but with physiotherapy and exercises have been able to improve their motor function enough to enable them to lead normal lives.

In old China, there was little care given to patients afflicted with polio. This was particularly so if they belonged to poor, working-class families. Recently, the Chinese have devoted much attention and research to treating these patients and claim to have achieved some miraculous cures. I was given an opportunity to visit children who were undergoing treatment in the traditional medical ward at Nanking Medical Institute. They were treated by acupuncture. None of the children admitted to that ward had ever had any form of treatment before. Now they receive physiotheraphy in addition to acupuncture.

The doctor in charge of the ward explained to me the rationale behind the treatment. He felt that they had found certain points on the body where acupuncture may produce stimulation of partially damaged or preserved nerve cells which may still be functioning. However, there was no scientific proof which could be demonstrated to us, nor were there any controls (patients who were just being treated with physiotherapy without any acupuncture).

But the children, as well as the medical workers, were very enthusiastic about the results. I met an eight-year-old girl who had been unable to walk prior to admission to the hospital. After six months of acupuncture treatment she was walking around without any help.

During a discussion on poliomyelitis, the doctor quoted Chairman Mao, "Qualitatively different contradictions can only be resolved by qualitatively different methods." The medical workers explained that the after effects of infantile paralysis differ widely from case to case because of the difference in the degree of damage, the site of damage, duration of disease, treatment received, and age. Each patient is placed in one of three categories for treatment:

1. Relaxed
2. Spastic
3. Mixed

Each of these receives a different grade of treatment—light for the first one—intermediate for the second one—intense for the third one.

Paralysis Resulting from Stroke or Head Injury

Although the Chinese claim that people with paralysis resulting from these conditions are improving with acupuncture treatment, I was not convinced. Some of the disabilities, I feel, improved on their own or sometimes with the help of physiotherapy.

One of the reasons for my skepticism in this situation is that the cells of the central nervous system, once damaged, do not regenerate. Any recovery of mobility that occurs is due to recovery of the function of temporarily or partially damaged brain cells, or because other areas of the brain take over the function of the damaged part.

This last switchover can occur much more easily in children. Once a part of the brain is lost, it is difficult to conceive how acupuncture could replace that loss. Acupuncture can effect the function of an organ, but once a part of that organ is lost, it cannot be compensated for by any procedure. What acupuncture accomplishes is the general toning up of a paralyzed extremity. However, it does not restore the voluntary control of movements. The same argument applies to the treatment of paraplegics.

Paraplegia due to Spinal Injury

At the Huashan Hospital, I saw patients with traumatic paraplegia. Their spinal cords had been damaged and they had total paralysis of their legs. They were being treated by acupuncture with electrical stimulation of the needles. I did not see any evidence of recovery of the function of their legs.

8

The Marvels of Acupuncture Anaesthesia

Acupuncture anaesthesia means using acupuncture as the sole method for relief of pain, while the patient is still awake. Its use in surgery, one of the most exciting innovations introduced in modern Chinese medicine, is a result of the integration of Western and Chinese medicine. I believe I was the first physician from North America to witness surgery under acupuncture anaesthesia. This was in June 1971. Since then many journalists and physicians have seen it and written about it.

Acupuncture anaesthesia was first performed in Shanghai in 1958. At that time, its use was suppressed by the then counterrevolutionary revisionist government headed by Liu Shao-chi (who was later deposed during the Cultural Revolution in 1968). According to the Chinese, some progress was made with this form of anaesthesia following the general policies outlined by Chairman Mao, "We cannot just take the beaten track transversed by the other countries in the development of technology and trail behind them at a snail's pace." However, it was not until ten years later, during the Cultural Revolution, that this form of anaesthesia became popular. Since then over 400,000 operations have been performed in China using acupuncture anaesthesia.

The general theory of acupuncture has been discussed in the preceding chapter. The same theories are used to explain the anaesthetic effect of acupuncture. The gate control theory of Melzak is still the most popular theory to explain this effect. The main gate, where the painful impulses are blocked, is in the dorsal (posterior) columns of the spinal cord. A second level where the painful impulses may be blocked is the thalamus, situated on each side, deeply in the cerebral hemispheres.

It is of interest that the most recent pain relieving device in neurosurgery, the dorsal column stimulator, uses the same gate control theory to explain its effectiveness. A pacemaker is implanted into the spine and is left in contact with the posterior columns of the spinal cord. Remote control electrical stimulation of this device inhibits the painful impulses at the spinal level and prevents them from reaching the brain.

Although the word "anaesthesia" is used very frequently the correct term is "acupuncture analgesia"—the second word meaning there's relief of pain. Anaesthesia means loss of sensations, but during acupuncture analgesia the patient does not lose the feeling of touch, only pain in the area of operation.

The Chinese have experimented on animals and noticed the electroencephalographic changes in certain parts of the cerebral cortex during acupuncture anaesthesia. These changes vary according to different points of needling. This infers that the effects of acupuncture anaesthesia are related to different levels of the central nervous system, with possible participation of other factors.

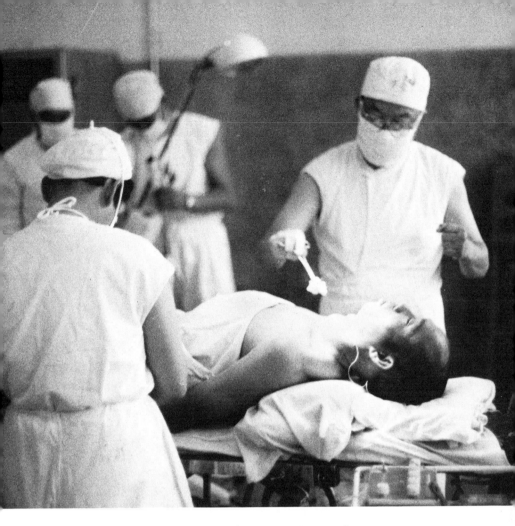

In this operating room scene,
the surgeon is cleaning the
patient's skin with the antiseptic
solution, Awete.

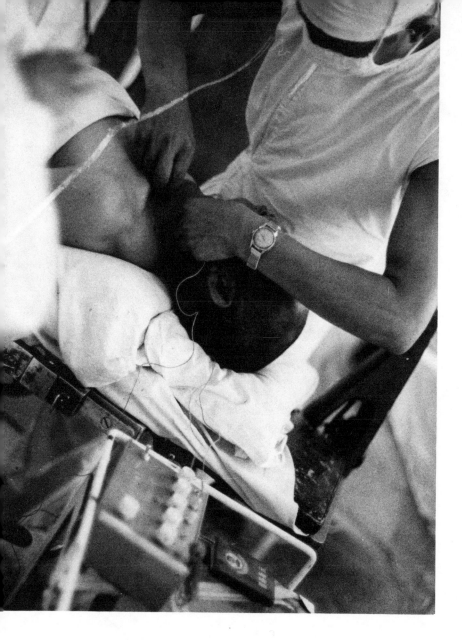

This patient is being anaesthetized with
acupuncture needles prior to a thyroid
operation.

No matter how it works, the Chinese continue to use acupuncture anaesthesia, and it is effective nearly 90 percent of the time.

Basic Technique

The patient is given a mild sedative the night before surgery. About one half hour before the operation is to take place, the acupuncture anaesthesia is started. The anaesthetist inserts stainless steel needles at the body's acupuncture points which affect the region to be operated upon. This usually corresponds to the traditional acupuncture points, although many new points have been added in recent years. The needle is connected to a direct-current, battery-power unit which delivers 6-9 volts, at 100-300 cycles per minute. In about one half hour, the patient is ready for surgery.

The stimulation is maintained throughout the surgery although the current varies according to the stages of the operation. During the part which may be very painful the stimulus is increased. It is dropped to a low level for the less painful parts of the procedure. Continuous stimulation for a long operation may lose its effectiveness. Sometimes no electric current is used, just the manual manipulation of the needle. But, generally electricity is used to save manual labor. In a long procedure with many needles, it would require more than one person to manipulate them. However, with the use of electronic gadgets all the needle stimulations on a patient can be controlled by one acupuncture anaesthetist. The needles are withdrawn before the patient is sent back to the ward but analgesic effects of acupuncture anaesthesia may persist in the post-operative period (from 24-48 hours). Some patients need further acupuncture, by manual technique, to relieve post-operative pain.

Operations Under Acupuncture Anaesthesia

I witnessed several operations performed under acupuncture anaesthesia. I will describe three of them:

1. At Huashan Hospital in Shanghai, I was taken to the operating room where many operations were being performed. Two of these involved brain surgery. One was on a young Chinese boy (age 14), who had a craniopharyngioma (a tumor situated at the base of the brain, above the pituitary gland). He had come to the hospital afflicted with headaches and progressive blindness. The diagnosis had been established and clinical examination done. Only a small x-ray of the skull had been taken. It showed some calcium deposited at the site of the tumor. Although the Chinese had all the special x-ray equipment available, they did not do any angiogram (x-ray of the skull after the injection of radiopaque dye into the cerebral circulation) and ventriculogram (x-ray of the skull after injection of air into the ventricles or cavities of the brain). This was purely an economic measure. x-rays are very expensive in China.

    Acupuncture anaesthesia had been started half an hour prior to surgery with three needles inserted —two on each foot and one behind the right ear. The patient, covered with surgical drapes, was fully awake and talking. An opening had been made into the skull on the right frontal region and two surgeons were removing the tumor when I arrived. I was able to look over their shoulders, see the tumor being taken out and even take photographs of the procedure. The surgical technique and dexterity of the surgeons was very impressive.

    A nurse acupuncturist administered the anaesthesia. She explained to me that she had started the stimulation from a nine volt battery at 120 cycles per minute, but during the time the incision was being made in the scalp (which is very sensitive to pain) the frequency was increased to 200 cycles. At the time the brain was being retracted to expose the tumor, the frequency was dropped again to 120 cycles and sometimes stopped altogether. This was done because brain tissue is insensitive to pain.

The procedure took two hours. Throughout this period the blood pressure, pulse, and respiration were monitored and remained quite stable. The tumor was completely removed. Since this was a benign tumor, the patient was expected to recover. At the end of the operation, the patient was able to get up and walk, with the help of an orderly, back to his ward. Hardly any loss of blood occurred and no blood transfusion was necessary because during surgery the bleeding points were coagulated with electric cautery (universal technique).

I asked the surgeon, Dr. Yu-Chuam-Shih, why he had been chosen to perform this operation. He answered that he is one of six neurosurgeons in the 56 bed department and explained that there is no chief in the department. All the neurosurgeons are equal and they are assigned cases depending upon each surgeon's experience and particular interest. They don't have problems getting along with each other. This particular surgeon had extensive experience in craniopharyngiomas, so he was assigned to this case. His assistant was a postgraduate trainee who was a general surgeon receiving six months' training in neurosurgery.

2.   This operation was also at Huashan Hospital and was a thyroidectomy on a 33-year-old woman who

had thyrotoxicosis. After the patient arrived in the operating room, there was a brief political discussion between the patient and the doctors. They quoted from the *Red Book* of Chairman Mao. This appeared to be a ritual after which the acupuncture anaesthesia was started with premedication of 50 mgm. Meperidine Hydrochloride. Two needles were used, one on the left wrist and one behind the left ear.

The operation was performed, in the usual way, through a neck incision and a portion of the thyroid gland was excised. Surgery went uneventfully and the patient, who experienced no pain, kept talking to the surgeon during the procedure. Later on, the surgeon explained to me the advantage of this technique, "When the patient is awake and talking this can prevent injury to the recurrent laryngeal nerve which supplies the voice box, thus preventing partial or complete loss of voice." The patient got off the operating table and without any help walked back to her ward. This is common practice.

3. At Bethune International Peace Hospital, I witnessed a pneumonectomy (lung resection for carcinoma). The patient, a middle-aged Chinese factory worker, had been a heavy smoker all his life. He had been admitted to the hospital a few days before the operation for tests, which included a chest x-ray, and also to learn breathing exercises, adopted from traditional Chinese medicine. Air had been injected into his right lung (the one affected with cancer) to collapse it. With exercises, the patient was able to adapt to breathing with the right lung collapsed and thus simulate the condition that he would face during surgery, when the right lung would collapse when exposed to at-

mospheric pressure from opening the chest wall.

Acupuncture anaesthesia was induced with only one needle to the right forearm. Later, additional needles were inserted to control the respiratory function. The most significant thing to me was that the operation was done without an endotrachial tube (a rubber tube placed into the main breathing passage). There was no positive pressure given. I found it difficult to believe that such a procedure could be done without endotrachial intubation. At that time, I was unable to get any explanation of this from the Chinese surgeon. Subsequent observation of similar operations and discussions with Chinese doctors gave me some idea of how this was possible.

In this particular case, the right side of the chest was opened and the lobe of the lung containing the tumor was resected. To avoid the mediastinal flutter (rapid to-and-fro movements of the structure in the mid-line between the two lungs) special acupuncture needles were used and stimulation was given. The patient was instructed to do deep abdominal breathing, thus lessening the movements of the lungs. He was fully awake during the procedure, talking, eating pieces of orange and having sips of water.

The operation took a little over two hours and went quite uneventfully. There was no blood loss and no blood transfusion given. The operative incision was closed after leaving a drainage tube and the patient was sent back to the ward in good spirits. Afterwards the surgeon explained that this technique had not been perfected. It cannot be used on a patient who has disease in both lungs and has poor pulmonary reserve.

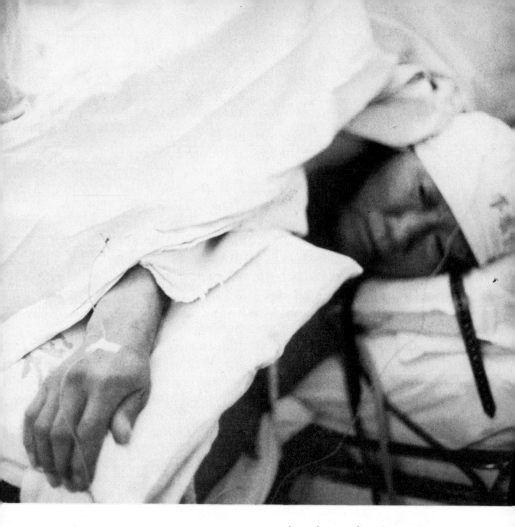

A patient undergoing surgery
under acupuncture anaesthesia.

Advantages of Acupuncture Anaesthesia

1. There are no major disturbances of physiological functions of the body like those that occur during the use of general anaesthesia.

2. There are no toxic effects.

3. There is no danger to life. No death has ever occurred from acupuncture anaesthesia. With general anaesthesia, there is still a mortality of about two per 100,000 operations.

4. The patient is awake and able to cooperate with the surgeon. This is of particular importance in surgery of the nervous system, when a surgeon wants to test the movements of particular parts of the body.

5. The period of recovery is short, the hospital stay is short, and postoperative complications are reduced.

6. The patient can eat and drink so there is no dehydration or electrolyte imbalance, which often occurs after general anaesthesia when there is a prolonged period of starvation.

7. There is no postoperative nausea or vomiting.

8. There are no postoperative respiratory complications.

9. There is no drop in the patient's blood pressure as there can be from general anaesthesia.

10. Adequate anaesthesia can be maintained for indefinite periods. This is of particular importance in

complicated procedures which may take as long as six hours. The intensity of electric stimulation is reduced during less painful parts of operations and increased during more painful procedures.

11. Surgery can be performed on critically ill patients and the very old or very young, who could not withstand general anaesthesia.

Limitations of Acupuncture Anaesthesia

Every patient cannot be operated on under acupuncture anaesthesia. There are some nervous and tense patients who decide against it. For them, the Chinese have facilities available for general anaesthesia. One of the brain operations that I saw in Shanghai was done under general anaesthesia. The patient had a tumor, situated very close to the brain stem, and any disturbance of that part of the brain would have caused respiratory arrest. During the operation, there was a tube inserted into the patient's trachia and he was on a respirator to control his breathing.

Abdominal operations are usually difficult as the abdominal muscles do not relax well under acupuncture anaesthesia, and during manipulation of the abdominal organs, traction can cause pain. Generally, operations below the level of the waist are difficult to perform under acupuncture anaesthesia.

Comparison of Western and Chinese Surgery

Surgery without general anaesthesia is not unknown in North America. A number of operations are still performed using a local anaesthesia, with the patient fully awake. In a few situations, hypnosis is used.

Spinal anaesthesia is sometimes used for operations on the lower part of the body. An anaesthetic drug is injected via a needle into the lower portion of the spinal canal. The type of operations which can be performed under local anaesthesia are rather limited. It is difficult to do major surgery without general anaesthesia. Very few patients are suitable candidates for hypnosis so this method cannot be adopted on a large scale.

The patient in North America who is given a general anaesthetic for a major operation usually has a longer stay in the hospital than a patient in China who has a comparable operation, for the following reasons:

1. Basically, the Chinese are very stoic people and tolerate trauma and surgery much better than the more sensitive North American patients.

2. An average Chinese is healthier than an average North American. The latter is usually obese and often has a number of ailments which make him more of a risk for an anaesthetic or an operation.

3. General anaesthesia has certain morbidity attached to it. Most patients do have aftereffects from it, such as nausea or vomiting. There is a recovery period of a few hours before the patient regains his full senses. This delays the patient's getting out of bed. In particularly prolonged procedures, followed by a long period of recovery from anaesthesia, the patient may be immobilized for a number of hours, this in itself can have an adverse effect on the body.

4. General anaesthesia creates a major stress on the human body. This, combined with the stress of

surgery itself, subjects the patient to double stress. Recovery is naturally more prolonged than if the patient had only one form of stress—surgery.

For the reasons outlined above, acupuncture anaesthesia definitely has an advantage. There are many situations where the number of operative complications are lessened if the patient is awake. During an operation many methods are used to assess a patient's condition. These measure blood pressure, pulse, and respiration, but they don't always give the true picture of the patient's health. If, however, the patient is awake, the important faculties of consciousness and power of speech can be assessed all the time. This assessment, combined with the patient's ability to carry out voluntary movements, can be of great help to a surgeon operating on the brain. Even in Western medicine, we see that the patient who has had surgery under local anaesthesia recovers much faster than the person who had similar surgery under general anaesthesia.

There are many other factors which influence the recovery of a postoperative patient. Most important is the patient's motivation to get better and his cooperation with the physician. This is seen at its best in China where patients have absolute faith in their physicians and are strongly motivated to recover. In North America, one encounters patients who are not fully confident in their physicians and those who have little drive to get well. These patients have a protracted recovery period following surgery.

Introduction of Acupuncture Anaesthesia into the West

So far, acupuncture anaesthesia has not been tried in Canada, but in March 1972 acupuncture anaesthesia was used at the Vienna Polyclinic when a tonsillectomy

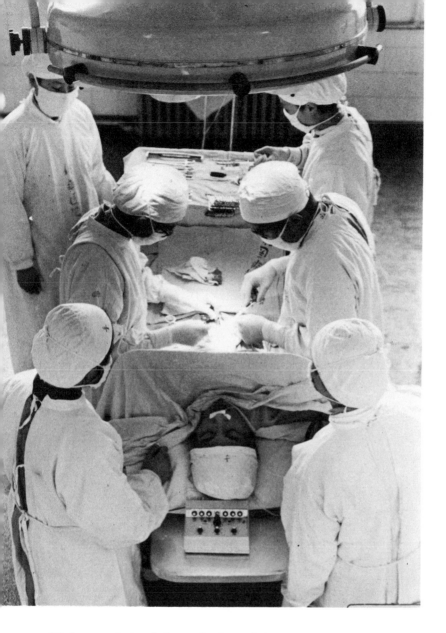

Modern surgical techniques also have their place in today's Chinese medical treatment.

was performed on a Viennese patient. Doctor Bischko, who gave the anaesthesia, had never visited China. He gathered his knowledge from reading reports of operations and studying books on acupuncture. The operation was quite successful. Doctor Bischko became the head of ENT Acupuncture section and has performed another twenty successful ear, nose, and throat operations under acupuncture anaesthesia. As of this writing he is planning to visit China for further studies in acupuncture.

In May, 1972 acupuncture anaesthesia was used in a New York hospital to anaesthetize a patient undergoing a skin graft operation. This is believed to have been the first in the United States. Since then a number of University Centers have started experimenting with acupuncture anaesthesia, but no conclusive reports on this have been published as yet.

Achievements of Chinese Surgery

Chinese surgery maintained high standards during the years when there was no contact with the Western world. Some of the achievements were:

1. *In the field of limb reattachment:*

According to Dr. Ha Hasien Wen, a Shanghai surgeon, a total of 321 of these procedures had been done in that city up to March, 1971. Out of these, 144 were for loss of fingers or toes. They had a success rate of 56 percent. Eighty-seven operations to replace arms or legs had a success rate of 82 percent. Some of these limbs were reattached as much as 36 hours after being severed, although Western doctors considered six hours the limit.

2. Open Heart Surgery:

The Chinese developed open heart surgery without much aid from the West. When the Russians were in China they planned to help the Chinese learn these techniques, but before this was accomplished they left. The Chinese built their own heart-lung machines and did open heart surgery under acupuncture anaesthesia with good results. However, they have not done any heart transplants.

3. Treatment of fractures:

In past years, the Chinese have followed the Western medical methods of treating fractures. They reduced the fracture and, if possible, immobilized the limb in plaster or applied traction. If the fracture could not be reduced, they operated and fixed the fracture with stainless steel plates and screws. In some cases a plaster cast was put on for two to three months. If the results still weren't good, immobilization and traction were prolonged, often causing bedsores and stiffening of the joints.

In 1958, under the guidance of the general line for building socialism, Chinese medical workers tried to combine Western and Chinese ways of treating fractures. Chinese traditional orthopedists were invited to demonstrate their methods. Over the next few years, it became clear that some of the traditional Chinese practices had the advantage of being simple, convenient, inexpensive, and effective. The traditional Chinese ways did not fit in with the Western concept of complete rest and extensive immobilization in treating fractures so there were objections to using the Chinese method of treatment. This opposition came mainly from the Western-trained Chinese surgeons. However, with the Cultural Revolution, further integration of the Chinese and Western methods resulted in China's present day approach to treating fractures.

Most fracture cases that I saw in the hospitals were being set with old-fashioned Chinese willow splints instead of plaster casts. This type of wood was selected because of its elasticity and strength. On the question of advisability of moving the limb after reduction, the Chinese traditional orthopedists have consistently favored immobilization coupled with appropriate movement. They quoted Chairman Mao "There can be no differentiation without contrast." There are two different ways of managing fractures and the results obtained from each were reviewed on the basis of prolonged clinical practice.

I was told that before 1958, when the Western method was used exclusively, it took 85 days for a fracture of the shaft of the femur (thigh-bone) to unite. After 1958, such fractures treated by a combination of Western and Chinese traditional methods, healed on an average of only 52 days, with good therapeutic effect. Clinical practice showed that a patient, bedridden for five to six weeks, lost one to two percent of his total bone calcium, even with the best nutrition. If the immobilization was prolonged, rarefaction of the bone (osteoporosis) occurred and bone union was delayed. With assimilation of Chinese traditional orthopedists' methods and summing up of patient's individual experiences, functional exercises were formulated which produced very good results in facilitating early union in fractures.

In addition, a number of herbal medications are used. How these medications work is not known and the effective constituents have not yet been isolated.

4. Treatment of Burns:

I mentioned in one of the earlier chapters, that there is a very famous unit for treatment of burns at the Nanking Medical Institute. As an introduction to the Chinese approach to burn treatment, we were told that the Chinese have applied dialectical materialist* theory of knowledge in treating burns and that they have been able to surmount difficulties and heal many serious cases, including babies and people well over seventy. They cited examples of cases where over 99 percent of the body surface was burned, 94 percent with third degree burns. By our Western standards such patients would not have much hope of survival.

They described their treatment of shock. This commonly occurs with severe burns because of the loss of blood and its constituents which leak out of blood vessels following the burns. Rapid pulse, a decrease in blood volume, a drop in blood pressure and other symptoms of shock follow. The patient may die if blood and saline are not given promptly.

The Chinese physicians used the Western approach to treatment of burn shock till 1958, but found that some patients did not improve. They therefore tried to find their own guidelines for the amount of fluid to be given. Urine output is now used as a guide to determine the amount of transfusions to be given.

After the shock is overcome, they concentrate on avoiding septicemia (infection of blood stream). Here again, they criticized the Western authorities who felt that germs can be dealt with in only two ways. One is to create a sterile field and the other is to use antibiotics to destroy the germs already in

*Reality, according to Marxism which views matter as the only thing subject to change. Change is considered the result of continual conflict which occurs due to the opposing forces present in everything.

the patient's body. The Chinese found that in many cases neither measure prevented septicemia. To overcome this situation, they combined traditional medicinal herbs and Western drugs, administering them, both by mouth and by local dressing, to increase the patient's resistance and aid wound healing. The necessary sterilization and isolation precautions were taken and antibiotics were used appropriately. The incidence of septicemia dropped markedly and the percentage of cure rose.

Plastic surgery is done on burn patients in China whenever necessary. They use a combination of autografts (taken from patient's own body) and homografts (taken from another person).

It is difficult to compare the Chinese methods for treatment of burns with the various units of the Western countries. There are some very good results being achieved in the United States and I feel that most of the burn clinics are treating patients adequately. However, the Chinese appear to be doing equally well and by utilizing the best of both systems of medicine. They have all the latest information about Western advances in the treatment of burns and they add this to the traditional herbal methods. Both patients and doctors seem very determined not to give up even in very serious burn cases. This determination is instrumental in salvaging many seriously-burned people.

Most of the cases of burns that we saw were from industrial accidents. As a matter of curiosity, I inquired about the safety precautions taken for industrial workers. Although the workers are provided with all the standard safety devices used in the West, they do not seem to use them. Because of this the number of industrial accidents, both burns and trauma to the limbs, is fairly high.

5. Brain Surgery:

The Chinese use Western techniques in their operating rooms. They have not used very many inventions or techniques of their own. One of the reasons for this is that the older Chinese neurosurgeons were trained in either North America or Russia and they are training the younger doctors in the same techniques. There isn't any definite residency training program as we have in North America. A neurosurgeon is trained, whenever one is needed, by attaching him to a neurosurgical unit. There is no fixed period of training and no examination is required. I did not see any neurosurgeons in training. At Shanghai Medical School Hospital, the only trainees I saw were general surgeons who were spending some time in neurosurgery in order to learn how to treat head injuries.

There are no figures available giving the total number of neurosurgeons in China, but there does not appear to be an excess of them. One of the largest departments of neurosurgery in China, Shanghai University Medical School, with 56 beds, had only six neurosurgeons. There was a tremendous amount of neurosurgery being done in this institute and, by American standards, it would appear understaffed. In a Western university department of that size, there would be at least three or four times the number of neurosurgeons, including the trainees. There are approximately 2,350 neurological surgeons in the United States.

An average neurosurgeon in the United States does not have a fraction of the important and complicated brain cases of his Chinese counterpart. Operative skill is largely dependent upon experience, and the Chinese neurosurgeons, in this respect, have the experience because of their limited number. This does not mean that they are short of neurosurgeons. No Chinese patient is left untreated because of lack of neurosurgical facilities and the neurosurgeons in China did not appear to be overworked.

The professional life of a Chinese neurosurgeon is far more interesting than that of an American neurosurgeon. He sees a variety of rare and difficult cases. But the private life of a Chinese neurosurgeon is lacking the luxuries enjoyed by the American. A busy neurosurgeon in North America is not necessarily busy doing surgery. He may be busy in research, teaching or in seeing office patients who have no surgical implications. Some neurosurgeons spend a great deal of time in courts testifying in medical-legal cases. The Chinese neurosurgeon is not implicated in legal action, which is a distinct advantage.

One striking difference between the practice of a neurosurgeon in the United States and one in China is the number of head and neck injuries he treats. Since there are few private automobiles in China, there are very few serious head injuries. In contrast some American neurosurgeons make their living almost entirely by treating victims of automobile accidents. If all these traffic accidents were eliminated, many Western neurosurgeons would find themselves unemployed.

Another difference is that a significant portion of the practice of a North American neurosurgeon is the treatment of spinal disc disease. Disc protrusions, both in the neck and the back, are very common in North America. In China, due largely to the Eastern posture of squatting, the incidence of disc disease is much lower. The number of patients in China who seek treatment from neurosurgeons is further diminished because many people get relief by traditional Chinese methods. During my stay, I did not see a single spinal operation being performed for removal of a slipped disc. One cannot go through a major North American hospital these days without seeing such an operation being done.

It is difficult to compare the neurosurgical morbidity and mortality of different countries. The Chinese, however, seem to be doing well, considering that their technical facilities are limited. They did not appear to have any more deaths or complications from operations than one might expect in such a serious type of surgery.

I was very impressed with the Chinese neurosurgeons. Watching them operate was a pleasure. They are adept at their work and know what they are doing. The Chinese neurosurgeon has the advantage of acupuncture anaesthesia which enables him to communicate with the patient during surgery. This makes the surgical procedure easier and the recovery of the patient is much shorter.

I observed a patient with a head injury who had regained consciousness, but was paralyzed on one side of the body due to brain damage. Since I was interested to know what plans the neurosurgeon had for rehabilitating this man I casually asked him what he planned to do about the paralysis. I was surprised when he told me that they were trying to cure him with acupuncture. Political indoctrination in China teaches the physicians not to accept any situation as hopeless. In a similar situation here, we would probably tell the patient that he would have to accept his paralysis because of the irreversible damage to his brain. We do the best we can to rehabilitate these patients, but we do not promise them cures. The Chinese doctors sometimes make statements which appear very unscientific to us, but it does appear to boost the morale of the patient.

I did not see any laboratory research being done by neurosurgeons. There was no evidence of the newer and more sophisticated techniques such as surgery under a microscope. In North America, most of the operations, particularly for repairing intracranial arterial aneurysms, (weak spots which can produce hemorrhage), are done under the operating microscope. The Chinese have these microscopes available, but they do not use them on a large scale. It was my impression that the Chinese prefer to get the information about new advances by reading the *Journal of Neurosurgery* (published in the United States). I did not encounter any situation where a neurosurgeon was dissatisfied with the present Western approach to neurosurgical problems.

The American neurosurgeons have the facilities and funding for research. Almost every university has a few interesting research projects going on. In addition to this, there are often facilities available for neurosurgeons in private practice to do research work. This appears to be essential as many of the problems in neurosurgery are unsolved at present. The standard techniques used for treatment of many conditions are unsatisfactory and there is a constant effort being made to improve on them and to find new methods. It appears the Chinese may step into the field of research in the near future, but whether they will have the same approach to it as we have is difficult to state.

I feel that soon neurosurgery, both in the East and West, will benefit greatly from the exchange of neurosurgeons between China and North America. The Chinese have some tremendously interesting clinical problems which the American neurosurgeons would like to see. The Chinese, on the other hand, could benefit from observing some of our newer neurosurgical techniques firsthand instead of just reading about them in our journals.

9

Herbs and
Modern Drugs

"Chinese medicine and pharmacology are a great
treasure house. Efforts should be made to explore them
and raise them to the highest level." (Mao Tse-tung)

Medicinal herbs are strongly emphasized in all
ancient Eastern systems of medicine. China has been one
of the largest growers of medicinal herbs. In old China,
herbs were not used selectively in treating diseases. Sometimes an herb was used to treat a particular organ, whose
shape or name it resembled. In those times, herbs were
found to be effective against certain diseases purely by
chance and their use continued and developed by trial
and error. As mentioned in the chapter on history of Chinese medicine, the *Materia Medica of Li-Shih-Chan*
(1518-1593) contained 12,000 herbal prescriptions. This
great work is still studied by the traditional Chinese physicians. As late as 1960 a Russian scientist selected 300 of
these prescriptions, subjected them to chemical analysis
and published his findings.

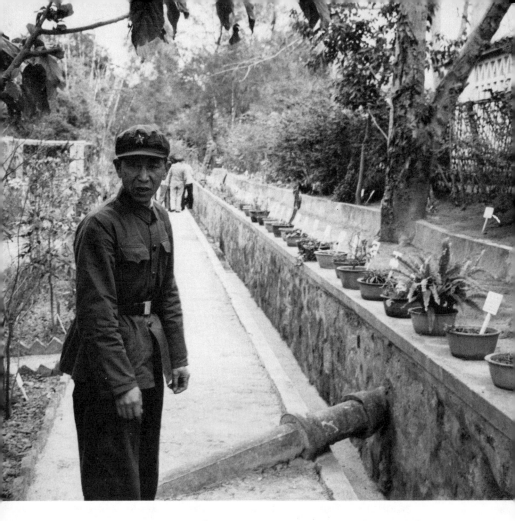

This elaborate herb garden is part of the military establishment. It is used to familiarize soldiers with herbs that may be eaten or used for medicinal purposes in the field.

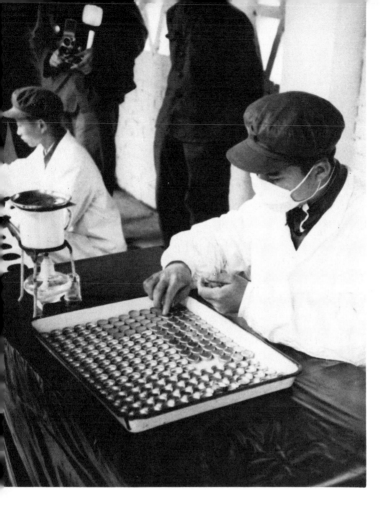

The soldier on the left is making mustard plasters while the other soldier fills containers with herbal ointment for army medical kits.

These Chinese patiently wait their turn to have prescriptions filled in a busy herbal pharmacy.

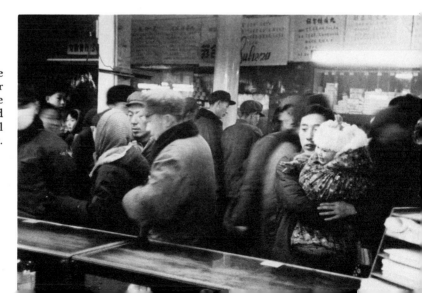

Everyone in China is a little bit of an herbalist. The housewives, the farmers, and even the school children grow herbs and learn to recognize them. Furthermore, herbs are easily available at stores, are extremely cheap, and are reasonably safe to use.

The medicinal power of a plant may be in its root, stem, bark, leaf, seed, or fruit. Various methods are used for preparing these medications. Sometimes just the dry plant is used, although it does not keep its strength in storage for long. One common method of administering Chinese herbs is by brewing them as a tea.

In ancient China, the use of herbs was accompanied by many rituals. The time of year, the time of day or night when the herb was collected, and the methods of preparation were of great importance. There were many religious and superstitious beliefs combined with the choice of herbs. Some of them were used as love potions. The use of love potions in modern China is almost non-existant and rituals have no place in modern medicine except for their psychological effect on those patients who are susceptible to suggestion.

Herbs in Modern China

Herbs have always been the main source of drugs for the traditional Chinese physician. During the regime of Chiang Kai-shek (1912-1949) the use of herbs declined along with the prestige of traditional Chinese medicine. Since the liberation of China in 1949, there has been a resurgence of interest in the herbs. It is impossible to list all of those which are in common use in China, but some of the better known ones are listed:

1. *The Ginseng (Panax Ginseng)*. This plant, whose roots are shaped like a man, is the Chinese

medicine best-known in the Western hemisphere. It is available in most Chinese drug stores in North America. This drug has maintained its reputation throughout the ages as a panacea for a host of unrelated diseases such as headaches, impotence, and rheumatism. Chemical examinations of this herb have not revealed any significant constituents which would explain its over-publicized beneficial effects.

2. *Chinese Horse Chestnut (Aesculus Chinensis).* This is used for rheumatism.

3. *Mugwort Wormwood (Artemesia Vulgaris).* Used in cases of severe diarrhea, menstrual disturbances and to stop blood spitting, this is also made into combustible cones and used in Moxa or cautery. (See next chapter).

4. *Senna Leaves (Cassia Angustifoba).* This is a popular laxative.

5. *Black Soya Bean.* This is ground and used for application on the skin to treat psoriasis.

6. *Chalmxoogra (Hydrocarpera Antehlmentica).* Oil extracts from this herb have been used as a treatment for epilepsy.

Various other animal and mineral herbs have been used. One of the best known is rhinoceros horn, which is powdered and used as an aphrodisiac as well as an antidote for poisons.

Trial of Herbs in Modern Hospitals

In various hospitals that we visited, clinical trials with herbs were being conducted to test their effectiveness on different ailments.

1. In the medical ward at Huashan Hospital in Shanghai, I saw a middle-aged Chinese who had been admitted after suffering a heart attack. He had high blood pressure and was being treated mainly with herbal medicines.

   A cardiologist with Western medical training examined him and had an electrocardiogram done. The patient was responding to the herbal medications. However, this treatment was combined with some Western medications, such as Papavrine (for dilating narrowed blood vessels to increase the blood supply to the heart).

2. We were shown patients with lung abscesses which were being treated with herbs. No modern antibiotics were used on these patients. Although the Chinese were unable to give us any exact statistics, they claimed they had successfully treated about 20 cases of lung abscesses without using antibiotics. They could not give us a detailed analysis.

3. Bacillary dysentery is treated with a combination of herbs and acupuncture.

Trial of Chinese Herbs in Surgical Conditions

1. *Treatment of Burns.*

At Nanking Medical Institute, which is well known for treatment of burns, modern surgical treatment of burns is combined with traditional Chinese medicine. Extracts of the leaves of Sophora Japonica (Japanese Pagoda Tree) and extracts of Aloe Sinensis (a variety of Aloes) were used for local application. The patients were treated by methods of exposure and the required skin grafts were performed by a plastic surgeon.

2. Gastric Hemorrhage.

One hundred-eleven cases were treated with herbs with a 70 percent cure. The average time required to stop the stomach hemorrhaging was 1.7 days, and the average hospital stay of a patient was 15.1 days. However, none of these patients had any barium x-ray studies to prove that they did have gastric ulcers. They also did not have any controls (patients with similar symptoms who were treated with no medications) in this study. It is difficult to compare this treatment with ours as we diagnose patients with gastric hemorrhage by doing x-ray study. Most of our patients improve with medical treatment.

3. Acute Abdominal Conditions.

Those on which surgery has traditionally been performed are being increasingly treated with herbal medications. The commonest one is appendicitis, for which the Chinese claim 80 percent success, and pancreatitis, for which they claim 90 percent success. They also report good results in treating cholecystitis and even ectopic pregnancies (pregnancies outside the uterine cavity). In all these conditions, the patients are watched very carefully and if they show no improvement with herbs, the surgeons operate.

4. *Cerebral Hemorrhage.*

I saw a young soldier at Bethune International Peace Hospital who had suffered a brain hemorrhage due to rupture of an abnormal communication between the arteries and the veins in the brain. The presence of blood had been verified by doing a lumbar puncture (insertion of a needle into the spine and removing the fluid from the circulation of the brain). X-ray studies, such as angiogram, had been done and showed the intracranial abnormality. However, the soldier was treated with bedrest and the use of herbs, which were supposed to reduce the chance of further hemorrhaging. He was subsequently discharged from the hospital. The surgeon told me he would operate if the patient returned with recurrence of his hemorrhage.

Research in Herbs

The Chinese are carrying out extensive research with herbal drugs. There are nearly 50 research institutes in China. These are some of the things they are investigating:

1. They are very interested in finding newer contraceptive drugs, and have tried hundreds of different herbs. Iris Palosii is considered one of the most effective. However, they have not had any proof of its success in clinical trials as yet.

2. They are looking for herbs with anticoagulant properties (preventing clotting of the blood).

3. They are testing herbs for anticancer properties. This appears to be quite a high priority in China.

Some of their other interests include finding herbal drugs for cardiovascular diseases and chronic bronchitis.

One of the biochemists whom I interviewed in the pharmaceutical laboratory of Peking University told me of the problems of research into herbs. He stated that sometimes the crude drug is effective against a certain condition, but when the contents are purified and isolated they are no longer effective. Maybe the process of brewing does something to the drugs; perhaps an essential factor is lost during purification.

Pharmaceutical Industry in China

China's pharmaceutical industry has developed quite rapidly. China is self-sufficient in all major drugs and even exports medicines to other countries. The national output of sulfa drugs, antibiotics, antidiuretics, anti-tuberculosis drugs, hormones, and vitamins has doubled since 1966 when the Cultural Revolution started. In spite of their increasing interest in the herbal drugs, the Chinese use all the modern antibiotics known in the West.

I was interested to know how the Chinese get antibiotics, but was unable to obtain precise information on this point. The Chinese do not import any antibiotics from Western countries. They are able to manufacture them in China. This is in keeping with Chairman Mao's teaching of "Maintaining independence and keeping the initiative in our own hands and relying on our own efforts."

In addition to increasing the supply of drugs, the Chinese have also been able to reduce the drug prices. At present, medicine costs only 1/5 of its price during the early postliberation period. The essential drugs such as vaccines, drugs for children, and contraceptives are supplied free of charge. In the Western world, we have a problem of high drug prices which are controlled by private enterprise. I was interested to note that in China drugs manufactured by students in pharmaceutical laboratories are not wasted but are marketed. The income from their sale is credited to the institution. These pharmaceuticals passed the quality control tests.

Pharmaceutical Research

The Chinese are very proud that they were first to determine the insulin crystal structure. This project started in 1958 and was a cooperative effort by the Institute of Organic Chemistry of Peking University and the Institute of Biochemistry in Shanghai. In describing their work, they quote frequently from Communist literature. They are told that the great teacher, Engels, pointed out long ago that "life is the mode of existence of albuminous bodies." As mentioned, this dialectical materialist conclusion is a most powerful criticism of metaphysical and idealistic religious beliefs.

Research work on protein is of great significance. The Chinese claim that, guided by Chairman Mao's revolutionary line, they were the first in the world to achieve total synthesis of biological active protein—crystalline bovine insulin by chemical methods in 1965. But, at that time, the basic structure of insulin and how it functioned was still not known. The work on this project continued even during the Cultural Revolution and x-ray crystallography was used to demonstrate the structure of insulin crystal. By January, 1971, the project was completed, nearly four years after it had begun. This work was quite independent of that being done in the United States, where similar results were obtained at about the same time.

It is difficult to judge the quality of pharmaceutical research in China, but the overall success in control of diseases cannot be ignored. They do not carry out strictly-controlled clinical trials with the precision of Western scientific methodology, but rely more on empirical observations.

10

Chinese Folk Medicine

In addition to acupuncture and herbs, there are many other methods of diagnosis and treatment in traditional Chinese medicine. They are briefly considered in this chapter.

Pulse Diagnosis

The pulse has always occupied an important place in Chinese medicine. A classic in this field is *Book of the Pulse* by Wang Shu-ho. Pulse diagnosis is still considered very important by physicians trained in the traditional Chinese way. The pulse is the rhythmic distension of the peripheral artery due to transmission of waves of blood flowing from the heart.

In our Western system of medicine, feeling the pulse of the radial artery at the wrist, and occasionally of the other arteries of the body, is a basic examination. It gives an idea of the rate of heartbeat. An abnormal pulse indicates the presence of disorders of circulation and occasionally of other systems of the body.

For the Chinese doctors, pulse diagnosis is an art in itself. Placing three fingers on the artery, they exert varying degrees of pressure. They do not feel just one artery but several arteries in different parts of the body. Diseases of internal organs as well as diseases of circulation are diagnosed this way in China.

According to the Chinese, there are twelve main pulses. Each pulse has some connection with an internal organ. Some of the pulses are deep enough to be connected with organs which are Yin (negative in character) and all the superficial pulses are connected to Yang (positive) organs. By examining the pulses they claim one can detect which meridian is at fault and subsequently track the defect to the organ. The Chinese prefer to take the pulse in the morning when they believe the Yin and the Yang are at rest. They would never take a pulse to test the stomach, liver, or gallbladder after the patient has had a heavy meal. Chinese acupuncturists say that there are twenty-seven pulses in all and that each of the main pulses can be subdivided to find further information about various parts of the particular organ shown at the pulse.

It is very difficult to find a modern, scientific explanation for this mode of diagnosis. Pulse diagnosis requires anywhere from 20 to 30 years of experience if one is to become an expert. Not very many physicians can wait that long to be able to diagnose ailments. Pulse diagnosis is also subject to a lot of errors. This has been verified when a number of physicians have tested the pulse of the same patient and each one has come up with a different diagnosis.

Although pulse has always been an important part of the clinical examination in Western medicine, and every doctor attaches some importance to it, I do not feel it is accurate enough to base a whole diagnosis on. One of the objects of pulse diagnosis is to locate the acupuncture points for treatment. It is much easier for a young physician to locate these points with the use of electronic devices than it is to depend upon pulse diagnosis. Therefore, I see very little prospect of pulse diagnosis becoming popular in the West. The modern Chinese physicians do not rely as much on the pulse as their predecessors, although they still have the traditional teaching in the pulse diagnosis.

Moxa Treatment (Moxibustion)

The word Moxibustion is derived from Moxa (Latinized form of Japanese plant Mogusa) and the Latin word bustum (a place where corpses are burnt). At one time burning herbs were applied at acupuncture points. Some of the older Chinese still bear scars from these burns. In modern China, this form of therapy is still in use, but now, instead of burning herbs, warm ones are used—the herb is crushed, wrapped in a special paper, held above the point to be warmed and then ignited. As mentioned in the last chapter the commonest herb used is Mugwort. Moxibustion is quite often combined with acupuncture.

It is difficult to explain the action of this form of treatment. Heat causes dilation of blood vessels of the skin and also stimulates some of the nerve endings in the muscles and blood vessels. The effect on the internal organ could be explained by the theory of referred pain since the area of skin is supplied from the same segment of the spinal cord which is receiving the painful impulses from the internal organs.

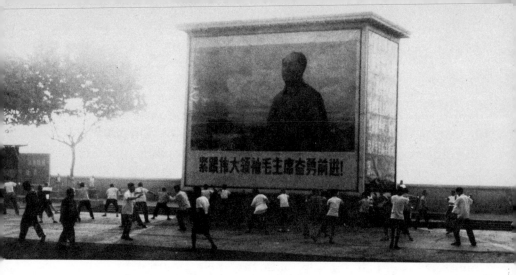

People performing T'ai Chi exercises before a poster of Mao.

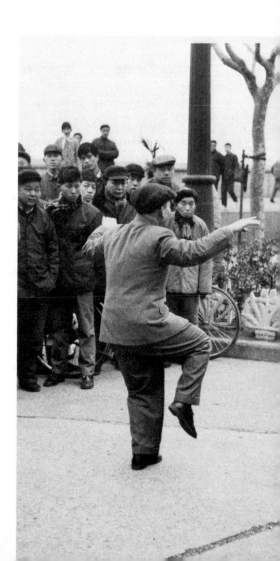

This elderly man is performing T'ai Chi, a type of exercise commonly practiced on the streets of China by people of all ages.

Physiotherapy

In traditional Chinese medicine, physical exercises are of great therapeutic importance and are also considered valuable in preventing disease. Most of the exercises originate from the so-called T'ai-Chi system. This is a very old system founded in the 10th century A.D. It is also based on the Yin and Yang theory and has some resemblance to the Indian system of Yoga exercises. T'ai-Chi consists of several hundred slow, coordinated, rhythmic movements performed in sequence by an individual or a group. The time taken to complete these exercises can be anywhere from one-half hour to one hour. They are usually done early in the morning or before going to bed.

I frequently saw T'ai-Chi exercises being performed in the streets very early in the morning. Although people of all age groups do these exercises, older people take part in them the most. Younger Chinese spend more time in modern sports, but they also do some modified forms of T'ai-Chi. The exercises are sometimes done using bamboo sticks or swords. The participants are supposed to abstain from smoking during the exercises.

The Chinese believe that these exercises help circulation and strengthen joints and ligaments. Physicians use them to supplement treatment of a variety of diseases, including high blood pressure, digestive disorders and some diseases of the nervous system.

Remedial Massage

This is a universal method of treatment for a variety of painful and debilitating conditions of the spine and limbs. In ancient China, the practice of massage was related to the practice of acupuncture. It was believed that massage of certain points could effect the function of the internal organs. The Chinese have a very elaborate system of remedial massage. Modern Chinese researchers are testing the efficiency of the ancient techniques, using equipment such as an acupuncture microamemeter.

In addition to the ancient system of remedial massage, the Chinese are also familiar with the Western system of physiotherapy. This is used in the treatment of hospital patients, particularly those who are paralyzed with strokes or injuries.

Breathing Exercises

Records show that breathing exercises have been a part of Chinese life at least as far back as the 5th century B.C. Like most Chinese theories the theory of breathing exercises is related to the Yin-Yang principle. These exercises differ from the breathing exercises of the Indian system of yoga. They are not simple inhaling and exhaling, but involve a complicated training program. There are many varieties of respiratory exercises. The Buddhists had their own system which was more related to religion and contemplation. It is believed that respiratory exercises can affect the function of the internal organs.

Modern Chinese research indicates that exhalation stimulates the parasympathetic part of the nervous system. This is used to explain why these exercises are prescribed for treatment of the autonomic nervous system. These respiratory exercises are commonly used to relieve a variety of disorders. However, the Western type of respiratory exercises are also used by the Chinese in the preoperative and postoperative care of surgical patients.

In conclusion, it may be stated that Chinese medicine uses many different breathing methods and one or more of them may be combined for any given patient. All these ancient methods are being investigated by modern Chinese physicians. Whenever they are found useful, they are incorporated into the practice of medicine. It doesn't matter whether their efficiency can be scientifically proven or not. To the Chinese, the important thing is whether or not a mode of treatment helps.

Comparison of Chinese Physiotherapy with Western Systems of Exercises

The basic difference between the Chinese and the Western systems of exercises is that the Chinese exercises are linked with philosophy. The Western system of exercises is purely physical. It is very easy to evaluate these exercises by the standard laboratory methods to determine their effect on the body. It is a little more difficult to evaluate the effect of the Chinese system of exercises, for example the T'ai-Chi, since there have been no scientific studies to measure body functions of a person doing T'ai-Chi exercises.

One may digress here and go to the Indian system of hatha yoga which is comparable to the Chinese system. At the All-India Institute of Medical Sciences elaborate studies have been done on yogis doing exercises. Some valuable scientific facts have emerged from these studies. It has been shown that a yogi can control his pulse and breathing and slow down his metabolic rate to a point where he could survive without oxygen for a much longer period than is commonly considered compatible with life. Electroencephalograms (brain wave studies) done during these exercises indicate slowing of brain activity and a state of ideal mental relaxation. Using this as an example, one can postulate that the Chinese system of exercises has a somewhat similar purpose in regulating the body. That the performers feel better after these exercises is beyond doubt.

In terms of effect on the heart and circulation, the most effective exercise is sustained physical activity, such as jogging or swimming. No other exercises achieve the physical effect on the cardiovascular system that these two exercises do. A person who jogs regularly and keeps in good physical shape has little chance of succumbing to heart disease, but he could have a nervous breakdown if his environment produces more psychological strain than he can handle. Conversely, a Chinese practicing T'ai-Chi may feel well and be able to maintain mental tranquility in spite of disturbing external environment, but he may die from heart disease.

The T'ai-Chi system of exercises does not have the same effect on the cardiovascular system as running. The ideal system of exercises is the one combining both. This is the reason for the resurgence of interest in the Eastern system of exercises in the United States. People have become interested in yoga and it is quite conceivable that they might also start learning T'ai-Chi just to obtain an optimal state of physical and mental health.

Other modes of physiotherapy (such as massage and respiratory exercise), are a very important part of the medical system in any country. In North America a lot of emphasis is placed on physiotherapy. Nearly every patient who has been in a hospital has had some exposure to these treatments. Massage, though done in different ways, is still used for muscular-skeletal disorders, and respiratory exercises are used for patients with respiratory diseases and to prevent lung complications after major surgery.

There is a mode of treatment comparable to moxibustion which was practiced, not too long ago, in the Western system of medicine. It has something to do with irritating the skin with the application of strong liniments. This is supposed to relieve pain by producing a reflex action in an internal organ. However, the Chinese moxibustion appears to be a bit extreme and it is unlikely that it will find much popularity in North America.

11

"Heal the Wounded, Rescue the Dying, Practice Revolutionary Humanitarianism"

(Mao Tse-tung)

It should be evident to the reader by this time that modern medicine in China is very heavily influenced by politics. During my visit to China, I noticed that political discussions dominate all medical conversations, both with individual physicians and members of a hospital staff. The same was true in conversations with the public as well as the patients. Most of the introductions to a medical conversation in modern China begin something like this:

"Under the guidance of Mao Tse-tung's proletarian revolutionary line and the cleansing fire of the great proletarian Cultural Revolution, a situation full of vigor and vitality has arisen on China's medical and health front. Armed with Mao Tse-tung's thought, medical workers have performed many miracles in medical work, writing a new chapter in the history of China's medical and health work."

Inadequacies of the Chinese
Medical System in the Past

The blame for inadequacies and failures in China's health field in the past are attributed to the influence of the deposed president of the Chinese People's Republic, Liu Shao-chi. This preceded the Cultural Revolution.

The explanation has the following implications: The failures are not seen as a result of technical deficiencies, but of incorrect political leadership. This explanation can be used to clarify situations where, in spite of massive allocations of resources in the Chinese Revolution, there were apparent medical failures. The explanation favors more social control of health workers and serves to prevent them from freeing themselves from it on the basis of technical expertise. It was believed that professional eminence made a doctor most vulnerable to the influence of Liu Shao-chi.

However, as Chairman Mao said, "Correct political and military lines do not emerge and develop spontaneously and tranquilly." Ever since the founding of New China, acute struggles have existed between the two lines of the medical field. Liu Shao-chi and his agents in health departments concealed themselves in the party, stubbornly pushing a counterrevolutionary revisionist line on health work, and making it serve only a few people.

They concentrated considerable manpower, material and financial resources on the urban hospitals, seeking to serve the *bourgeoisie*. They turned the medical and health departments into revisionist's hot beds for their own survival. No attention was paid to the common, recurrent diseases most harmful to the masses. These opportunists attempted to lead the people's health work down the capitalistic road. Thus they committed towering crimes against the people.

The great Proletarian Cultural Revolution completely smashed Liu Shao-chi's plot to restore capitalism. The working class (the main force of the Proletarian Cultural Revolution) and the poor and lower-middle class peasants have mounted the political stage of struggle in response to Chairman Mao's directive, "The working class must exercise leadership in everything." Putting Mao Tse-tung's thoughts in command of everything else, they have brought about a great change in health work.

Political Ideology as a Guide to Treatment Priorities

The following quotations from Mao Tse-tung are pertinent in the discussion of this topic.

1. "This question 'for whom?' is fundamental; it is a question of principle." In a class society medicine serves a particular class—in modern China it should be placed at the service of all people.

2. "Vigorous action should be taken to prevent and cure endemic and other diseases among the people and to expand the people's medical and health services."

3. "In medical and health work, put the stress on rural areas."

4. "Of the two contradictory aspects, one must be principal and the other secondary. The principal aspect is the one playing a leading role in the contradiction. The nature of the thing is determined mainly by the principal aspect of the contradiction, the aspect which has gained a dominant position."

The political ideology affects the health-care system in the following ways:

1. It provides for a disease to be evaluated in an entirely new way, using new techniques. For example, neurasthenia is treated by daytime excitation and nighttime relaxation.

2. It motivates medical workers to overcome the failings of previous clinical knowledge and their own lack of experience and training. It does not forbid them to make use of Western scientific knowledge, although the Western political philosophy is condemned.

3. It is used as a motivational device to help medical workers to deal with emergencies.

4. It leaves room for laymen to make medical discoveries.

5. It puts the emphasis on medical care in the rural areas, where the majority of the population lives.

In response to Mao-Tse-tung, thousands of revolutionary medical workers left modern buildings in the city for the rural and mountainous areas. They settled among the masses, accepted re-education by the workers, peasants, and soldiers and sought to serve them. It is estimated that 300,000 urban medical workers moved to rural areas and another 400,000 made trips to the countryside.

The Chinese health care system is not governed internally, but is influenced by the external political system. This minimizes the build-up of a professional hierarchy organized around technical expertise or seniority. In this system, where a clear-cut distinction between doctors and nurses cannot be maintained on the basis of their efficiency, a doctor who is technically expert, but political-ly naive may be at a disadvantage.

The Rationale of the Political Role in the Reorganization of Health Services

The following points illustrate the reasoning be-hind the modification of the medical system instituted by political influence to suit the best interests of the country:

1. Because there are so many rural areas, all the tech-nical equipment devised has a portable version that can be transported to remote parts of the country to serve the sick. This is more desirable than wait-ing for the patient to be transferred to the city. At the Shanghai Industrial Exhibition, I saw portable models of all the important diagnostic tools, in-cluding electroencephalogram, X-ray machines, and echoencephalogram (diagnostic tool for the brain using ultrasound). Even the most so-phisticated surgical instruments were designed to be put into carrying cases, which a surgeon can take in his handbag, thus enabling him to perform surgery in a small hospital with limited facilities.

2. There is emphasis on preventive health care and early treatment. This has been achieved mostly by the mass movement inspired by political change. It has, in turn, cut the cost of health care and drastically reduced the epidemic diseases.

3. The use of paramedical personnel has led to better treatment in areas where qualified doctors are not available. It also provides a better liaison between the doctors and the patients, as the lay medical

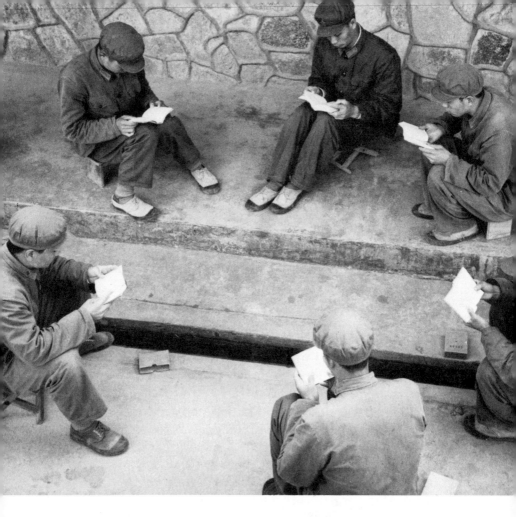

Reading from the works of
Chairman Mao is a standard
part of all meetings.

workers are from the communities they serve and understand the social environments.

4. Health care is provided with an awareness of the sociopolitical needs of the patient.

5. The hospital health workers must frequently leave their hospital base and take up duties in the countryside, providing health care directly for those who find it inconvenient or impossible to come to the hospital.

Ideology as a Motivational Device for Health Workers and Patients

Health workers often encounter situations where they have uncertainty, fear, or clinical ignorance of a particular diagnosis or treatment of an apparently incurable disease. These sources of tension are reduced by political indoctrination. Time and again, I encountered descriptions of medical treatment where either paramedical workers or physicians, encountering a difficult situation, referred to Mao Tse-tung and one of his often quoted statements, such as:

"Be resolute, spare no sacrifice and surmount every difficulty to win victory."

"Man has constantly to sum up experiences, go on inventing, discovering, creating, and advancing."

Such political indoctrinations do serve their purpose in helping overcome fear in the medical worker. Every hospital has a Mao Tse-tung propaganda team and one of their tasks is to motivate health workers by reading them passages from Mao. This ideology prevents the health workers from getting too conceited about their successes.

The same ideology also works as a motivational device for patients. The rationale for this is that social control over an individual is at its lowest when he is sick and the patient can then claim exemption from normal requirements. The Chinese health care system surrounds hospital patients with portraits of Mao and placards bearing his sayings. This is aimed not only to maintain social control by reasserting the bonds of collective loyalty even in sickness, but also to motivate the patients to get well and resume active roles. Loyalty to Mao is defined on the patient's part as a belief in the "curability" of his ailment, in proper cooperation with health workers, and there is a feeling of optimism and courage about the medical outcome. Both health workers and patients are helped in dealing with feelings of personal inadequacies, fears, and uncertainty, by the behavioral guidelines derived from Mao's thoughts. This is achieved by complete penetration of the health system by ideologies of Chairman Mao, which relates the most technical details of their system to the wider political goals of the society.

Comparison with the American Health System

It would appear futile to compare the American health system with the Chinese health system in view of the political indoctrination outlined in the previous pages. There are three important factors in the American case which prevent any influence on it by the wider cultural values of society, and these are:

1. Lack of ideological concensus among many diverse political philosophies.

2. Professionalism. This implies that there is a private

informational system language used by system members.

3. Private medical practices.

None of these three factors are present in modern day China. The American physicians are studying the Chinese health care system and some points could be adopted which would improve the medical care in the United States. The following are possibilities and in no way definite recommendations:

1. America could serve needy rural areas and decentralize the medical services in the cities.

2. We could create a large paramedical force in the rural and industrial sectors of the population to provide a better primary care for working people.

3. Our government control could be increased and a more comprehensive health care system created. At present, the medical care controls are vested in different organizations at different levels. Even the Medicare program for the aged is not comprehensive enough.

4. We could improve health services for the underprivileged members of the society. This could be best done by a state controlled, prepaid comprehensive medical care plan, covering both medical care and hospitalization at a cost which the poor people could afford. Those who couldn't afford to pay the premium for such a service should be subsidized by the government. Discrimination in treatment, based on economics, will have to be abolished to remove the disparity in the standard of patient care between underprivileged and privileged segments of society.

We can aim for a better patient-physician relationship in the North American society by eliminating some of the barriers. The Chinese political philosophy holds everyone on an equal status so the doctor feels much closer to the patient. Doctors treat patients as a matter of service and not as a business with financial rewards. In China, due to increasing participation of lay people in the health field, there is no mystery in medicine.

Role of Political Indoctrination in Determining Success of Medical Aid to Underdeveloped Countries

The United States has been heavily involved in giving medical aid to underdeveloped countries all over the world. This has been done primarily in two ways:

1. They take students, mostly at postgraduate level, from underdeveloped countries and provide them opportunities for training in the United States. The goal is for these students to go back and improve the medical care in their own country.

2. They provide financial aid.

Both these methods usually fail. Most of the students who come to the United States stay after completion of their postgraduate studies. They find it difficult to work in a primitive country after being trained in a very sophisticated medical environment. The financial aid seldom goes to the segment of society that needs it. Most of it ends up in the hands of profiteers in the under-developed countries, and the benefits never reach the general population. My reason for pointing this out is not to criticize the American system, but to give an example of how China carries out a similar activity.

In 1969, the Chinese sent medical teams to Yemen. Earlier Soviet doctors and Western European doctors had tried to accomplish this mission unsuccessfully. The Chinese sent medical personnel who worked directly with the people. They did a lot that was useful and earned the gratitude of the people of Yemen. The people they treated were the type who had been neglected by the Russian doctors, or were considered incurable by the Russians and given no assurance or encouragement in their hopeless illnesses.

In the same year, the Chinese carried out a successful medical-aid mission in Algeria. The Chinese claim that their health system is vastly superior to those of Russia and the Western countries in terms of medical assistance to such underdeveloped countries as Yemen and Algeria. The usual example given is that Russians or Western clinical authorities declared cases incurable which were later cured by the Chinese. The difference is that the Chinese teams are armed with Mao Tse-tung's thought and are thereby endowed with political and social awareness of the needs of the peasants that they treat.

12

Some Observations About Chinese Medicine

My visit to China was fascinating and educational. The history of Chinese medicine that I had studied was very much alive in modern China. Their health care was better organized and of a higher level than I had anticipated for a populous Eastern nation. Our hospitable hosts did all they could to provide me with the information that I was seeking. However, there were limitations and I was unable to see everything that I wanted to. There were certain topics that the Chinese avoided. Under these circumstances anything written about China becomes more of an individual's own impressions than statements of the actual facts. Statistics are very difficult to come by, as some of them have not yet been compiled, and an average doctor in China is not much concerned with the national statistics about a particular disease.

One of the most striking things about Chinese medicine was the political overtone. There was hardly any medical discussion which was not preceded by political discussion and quotations from Mao Tse-tung. The Chinese believe, and to some extent they are right, that most of their medical progress is a result of the political leadership provided by Mao Tse-tung. However, this point is often carried too far, such as recitation of Mao's quotations prior to the start of a surgical operation. This appeared more like a religious ritual than a scientfic treatment.

Some physicians were less than frank in their discussions with us, due to the presence of nonmedical politicians in the medical institutions. For example, the Revolutionary Committee of Nanking Medical Institute had as their spokesman a non-medical man who monitored the conversations between the medical staff and us. There were many questions which they did not want to answer and they were completely omitted in the translations made by their interpreter. Although some of the physicians could speak English, they preferred not to talk to me directly in English, but rather in Chinese through the interpreter. Then everyone present, including the nonmedical politician, could listen to what was being said. There were some problems as some of the non-medical people could not quite understand some of the medical problems which we wanted to discuss. In China, medicine is everyone's business and everyone is supposed to be capable of discussing general medical problems. In the West, medicine is considered very technical and any discussion on medical problems is the domain of specialists in this field.

The other outstanding thing about Chinese medicine is the emphasis on preventive medicine. This type of emphasis is not easy in any country where medicine is a private enterprise. However, China has somewhat of a socialized system of medicine. The doctors are more interested in preventing disease than spending their time treating it. Some of the greatest advances made in modern

China are in the field of preventive medicine. Their conquest of the epidemic diseases and the venereal diseases is a monumental example of the group effort of a socialized state guided by the unified political philosophy and selfless attitude of the people. In this respect, we rather envy the Chinese. In spite of their lower material standards, they have higher health standards than most of the Western countries. Venereal disease has become quite a problem in North America and it is still on the increase. We have drug problems and we still have a lot of infectious and epidemic diseases, particularly in some of the less privileged segments of our society. In solving these problems, we may have a lesson to learn from the Chinese.

In medical economics, the West is faced with the problem of spiraling medical costs. It seems that all the material wealth of North America, both in the United States and Canada, is insufficient to keep up with the rising cost of medical care. The Chinese have kept this problem in the background a number of ways, such as socialized medicine with no private enterprise and a guarantee of medical care for every citizen. In addition to this, the integration of the traditional and modern systems of medicine has reduced medical costs. This union had more than sentimental reasons behind it. There was a potential manpower in China with medical training which was being wasted. Integrating the two systems enabled the Chinese to utilize all their medical manpower. Another way they lowered the cost of medical care was to create the barefoot doctors. Although these people do not get paid as much as physicians, they do the sort of work that constitutes about 50 percent of an average general physician's practice in North America.

We are still experimenting with the idea of physician's assistants. The Chinese have already implemented this on a nationwide scale and have proven it to be a sensible, cheaper way of providing primary medical care. It fits very well with the Chinese philosophy and their way of life at the present time. Our North American public would not be fully satisfied if the care were provided by anybody not having the title "M.D." I personally feel, that for minor ailments and disorders, we should utilize all the available medical manpower to do the primary treatment of patients. It is very important, however, that this be done under the guidance of qualified medical doctors. This is the case in China, where a barefoot doctor refers his patient to a regular doctor if he feels that the patient's ailment is no longer minor.

Acupuncture, of course, has caught the fancy of Western nations. This sudden interest is incomprehensible to the Chinese who have had acupuncture for thousands of years and have been using it as a form of anaesthesia since 1968. The Chinese doctors are surprised that some Western physicians are enthusiastic about acupuncture anaesthesia and are flocking to China to see it. They seem indifferent to the criticism of the skeptical Western physicians who believe that acupuncture anaesthesia is some hokus pokus or a form of hypnosis. Although the Chinese have not been able to give us an explanation of the mode of action of this form of anaesthesia in our own scientific terminology, they have continued to use it successfully on thousands of patients. For them all that matters is that it works for the majority of the patients. They are not against sharing their discoveries and information. They are simply waiting for the required proof that this form of anaesthesia works before submitting their findings for publication in the West.

One reason for the lack of publications on medicine in the past few years has been the peculiar Chinese attitude towards research and publications in general. This was again influenced by political changes of the

Cultural Revolution. It is not considered desirable for a doctor to seek fame by doing research and publishing a paper. He was supposed to devote all his time to serving the people by practicing medicine. Some very high-powered medical professors were sent to work in the fields with farmers so that they could regain their sense of identity with the people and learn to think of medicine in a practical rather than an academic manner.

The whole Chinese approach to medicine can be illustrated by the following example. Supposing a patient has pain in the stomach and is seen by the barefoot doctor in the patient's community; he tries herbs and acupuncture and if the patient does not get well he is referred to the clinic or hospital to be investigated by a fully-trained doctor. The doctor tries to rely on a clinical diagnosis and use herbal treatment before proceeding to more complicated investigations such as specialized x-rays. Thus, surgery is avoided if at all possible and is used only as a last resort.

In contrast to this, a patient in the West with the same sort of problem can go directly to a specialist and have the most expensive and sophisticated tests done. Often nothing is found to be wrong. The total cost of examining such a patient can run into hundreds or thousands of dollars. Some patients are not satisfied with the opinion of one specialist and go on to another. Finally, some of them end up having unnecessary surgery. Such things do not happen in China. The Chinese cannot afford it.

There is no such thing as cosmetic surgery in China. The people are not very conscious of appearance. They are proud of being Chinese and want to look Chinese. Nobody wants to go and have the shape of their eyes or nose altered to make them resemble the Caucasians.

Medical exchanges between China and the Western

countries are still very limited. The Chinese are not too anxious to have tourists or visiting doctors come, although they are proud to show their work and the development of some of their newer techniques, such as acupuncture anaesthesia. They are, however, interested in visiting the Western countries and at the time of this writing we are expecting a Chinese medical delegate to visit us.

The Chinese general way of life is very clean, orderly and well regulated. It consists of work, sleep, and physical exercises. The people are well fed but I seldom saw anybody who was obese. The children, particularly, are in excellent health. About the only bad habit that I noticed was smoking and that is gradually being curbed. The children and armed forces personnel are not supposed to smoke. However, on a few occasions, we saw some members of both these categories smoking. They were severely rebuked by other Chinese who happened to spot them. This is in keeping with the Chinese way of self-discipline. In our society, few people point out to another individual what he should or should not do. But in China it is not considered impolite for someone to tell another person that what he is doing is not good for him or society. Obviously such a society does not need many preachers or policemen. They have a built-in system of discipline due to very strong political indoctrination right from early childhood.

This has its advantages and disadvantages, but, from a health point of view, a person who has been well disciplined from his earlier days is likely to be healthy. However, the Chinese in high positions are not immune to the stresses and strains of life and are subject to the same sort of illnesses that happen to people in high positions in the Western society.

A harmonious and cooperative spirit prevails between the various categories of medical workers. The patient takes part in discussing his problem. The prescription given to him is in the language that he can read (in contrast to the Latin prescriptions written by some of the Western physicians) so that he knows what he is taking. Chinese doctors believe that this frank attitude with their patients improves the chances of successful treatment.

13

The Future of China and Chinese Medicine

"It is only 45 years since the Revolution of 1911, but the face of China today is completely changed. In another 45 years, in the year 2001, China will have undergone even greater changes. She will have become a powerful, socialist, industrialist country. And that is as it should be." (Mao Tse-tung, 1956)

China already has become a major world power, in industry, agriculture, and nuclear power. With the recent admission of China to the United Nations, China's role in the world has assumed great importance. The question now being raised is: What will China be like in the year 2001?

Will Chinese progress continue, or has it already reached a peak? The same question could be asked about the United States. Has the peak of modern civilization been reached and is it going to decline as it has in all past great civilizations? It is very difficult for futurologists to predict.

Anticipated Advances in Medicine in the Western Countries by the Year 2001

We expect advances in the following general areas:

1. The possible cure of cancer.

2. Genetic engineering of the human body. This will mean modifying the genes to eliminate undesirable traits.

3. Mechanical organs, such as a mechanical heart.

4. Electronic devices to replace damaged parts of the nervous system. This might include replacement of portions of the brain to help people with paralysis from strokes. This might solve the problems of paraplegics.

5. Automation of medical procedures such as patient records, history taking, laboratory tests, and diagnosis. This is already being instituted in some of the American hospitals.

6. Cure of some of the poorly-understood diseases.

Future of Chinese Medicine

The evolution of medicine in China is continuous, like the social revolution, and it will likely result in better care of the masses. By the year 2001 China will have eliminated most of the epidemic diseases and significantly increased the life span of its population to bring it within comparable figures of life expectancy in the Western nations.

The resumption of medical education and research in China will have some dramatic effects in rasing the standards of medical care (which is by no means low now). We can foresee the resumption of publications of Chinese medical journals and books and more exchange of medical personnel and information between Chinese and Western nations.

The impact of such an exchange will be significant to the practice of medicine in Western nations, particularly North America. It is likely that the use of procedures from Chinese medicine will be adopted and integrated into the practice of Western medicine.

Further research into acupuncture and its efficiency as an anaesthetic is needed. It would not surprise me to see acupuncture anaesthesia replace general anaesthesia in North America. This, however, will not be an easy transition and will take time.

Pharmaceutical research into ancient herbs is bound to be of use. Perhaps a drug will be found for a disease presently considered incurable. It is possible that the application of sophisticated laboratory techniques, developed by the pharmaceutical companies in the United States, could make significant contributions to the refinement of active ingredients of some of the ancient herbs.

The economics of the Chinese Medical Organization is a good example for other underdeveloped countries. As a matter of fact, there is something to learn even for the richer nations of the West. No country is rich enough to keep up the rising cost of medical care. The overmedicated society in North America may get rid of some drugs after a careful study of the Chinese system of medicine.

At the time of writing this book, two states—California and Washington, have permitted the practice of acupuncture as an investigative procedure under supervision of M.D.'s in university medical centers. The Province of British Columbia is investigating the possibility of licensing acupuncturists. It is likely that the practitioners of Chinese medicine will be able to serve the public so long as this service is done with the approval, and under the supervision, of M.D.'s. This appears to be in the best interest of the public.

14

My General Impressions of China

I noticed a marked contrast on crossing the border into China. It was like stepping into a new world. Street beggars and the wealthy-looking, Western-type Chinese were conspicuous by their absence. We saw scantily dressed farm workers proudly toiling in the fields, doing most of the work with their hands. Occasionally we saw some farm animals, plodding along helping the farmer, but there were no heavy agricultural or mechanical machines. Although the Chinese manufacture tractors, they have been slow to mechanize. At the present time, there is no unemployment in China.

The Chinese people work extremely hard. Their usual working day is supposed to be eight hours, but I saw farmers starting work as early as 6:00 a.m. and continuing to work until 6:00 in the evening. Many people work overtime both in the fields and the factories, not for any extra pay, but simply to show that they have good motivation. In some places commune members are competing with other communes for higher agricultural-output figures. The hard working Chinese are exceptional people in the Eastern world where farm workers take long siestas, particularly in the summer. I never saw a Chinese taking a nap in the field during the middle of the day.

The only time I encountered someone sleeping on the job was while I was riding a street bus. The conductor was asleep when I wanted to pay the bus fare and he would not wake up. Another passenger, a young girl of about thirteen, woke him and admonished him for sleeping on duty. This is typical of the Chinese disciplinary system which is controlled by the people themselves and not forced on them externally by police. Every citizen has the right to criticize another person openly for any breech of discipline. I saw another example of this when a purse-snatcher was apprehended by bystanders in Peking. This was the only incident of theft I saw in China. After the offender was apprehended he was rebuked by the citizens and then allowed to leave. There was no arrest made and we were told that these petty cases seldom go to court.

One of the most outstanding features of Chinese life is discipline. It is instilled in the people from child-hood. For a society built on revolution, where revolution is considered a perpetual state, the Chinese are indeed very well behaved. The basic disciplinary organization on the community level starts with a block mother. This is usually a middle-aged housewife, responsible for main-taining discipline in one residential block. I saw the disci-plinary organization in action when the children crowded around our group, their curiosity overcoming their sense of discipline. The block mother was not able to handle the situation and had to call in the next highest neighborhood authority who was a cadre and held Communist Party membership. He tried to talk the children into going back to their homes while the block mother diverted all traffic

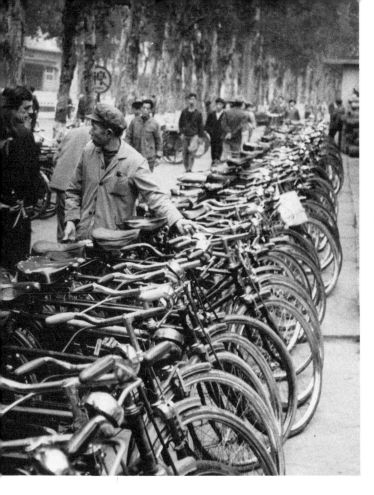

Bicycles are the most common form of transportation in China.

away from the crowded area. With a system like this, a large police force is unnecessary.

The only policemen I saw were those guarding important state buildings and those controlling the city traffic at busy intersections. Cars, buses and pedestrians crossed these intersections wherever they wished in spite of the bullhorn reminder by the policeman not to go against a red light. No one was given a ticket for jaywalking and since there are very few automobiles there are not many accidents. The private ownership of cars is forbidden in China and the few cars on the road belong to the government and are used to transport people on official business. In spite of this, the Chinese get where they want to go. There is good public bus service available and most of the citizens also ride bicycles. Peking (with seven million population) has a very modern subway system which had just been completed at the time of our visit. We were given a demonstration ride through this subway which is also designed to serve as an air-raid shelter.

Transportation to work is seldom a problem as most of the people live within a short distance of their place of employment. There are no real traffic problems, in spite of the huge population of China and the large number of inhabitants in the large cities. I don't think the Chinese realize how lucky they are to be deprived of private auto ownership and avoid the problems of traffic congestion and air pollution that we have in North America. We are just beginning to walk and ride bicycles for health reasons. In China these things are a way of life.

Honesty

The Chinese honesty was evident in every walk of life. As a traveler who has been cheated in business transactions in Eastern bazaars, I found this a surprising relief. The prices of things were fixed and no haggling took place. It is considered fair game throughout most of the East to charge exorbitant prices and fleece the rich, North American tourists. In China prices are reasonable.

No traveler loses anything in China. There are countless stories of people getting things back, even when they wanted to get rid of them. The individual Chinese does not accept handouts, tips, or gifts. One journalist tried to leave a pen, but it was traced to him and delivered to him at the border before he left the country. I lost a pair of socks in a laundry—two weeks later they caught up with me in another city. One of my colleagues on the tour forgot to get back two cents change from a bus conductor.

Four hours later the conductor traced him to our hotel, approached him in the hotel lobby and returned the two cents. The man had taken several hours locating the hotel and finding my colleague.

Most hotel room doors have no locks and we left our valuables, including photographic equipment in our unlocked rooms. However, we did notice that a lot of bicycles had locks on them. This seemed somewhat inconsistent, so we inquired about it. One of the bicycle owners explained to me that this is to prevent other people from mistakenly taking the wrong bicycles since most of them are the same make and look alike. Some skeptics say that the Chinese don't steal anything from Westerners for fear of being detected and because they would not have much use for Western things. I am personally convinced that the Chinese are basically honest.

Clothing, Women and Fashion

The Chinese dress very simply. Both men and women wear drab-colored, plain shirts and baggy pants with the cuffs rolled up and the ankles showing. Quite often they go barefoot. The pretty Chinese women don't look very elegant in these clothes or army uniforms, but there is a certain charm in their simplicity. It is not acceptable to use many cosmetics or to enhance one's sexual attractiveness by dress. Only the children are dressed colorfully. The Chinese are essentially a puritanical society.

It is quite common to see Chinese women wearing rubber bands on pigtails. They use no fancy hair ribbons and seldom wear nailpolish or lipstick. They do not seem envious of Western women who visit China wearing fancy clothes and makeup and the Chinese men disapprove of Western women who wear mini-skirts and low-cut dresses.

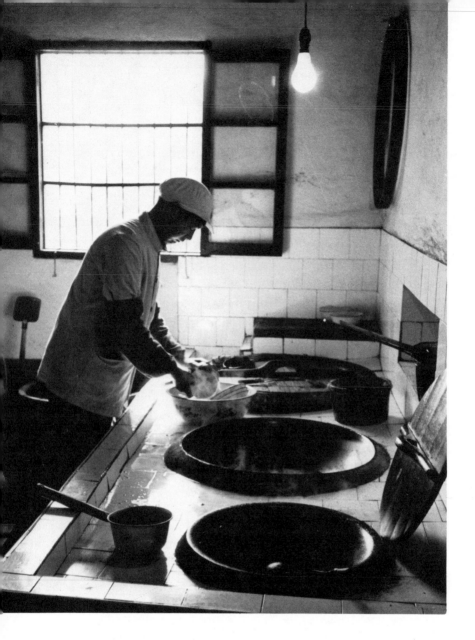

This cook is preparing food in
a commune kitchen.

The common Chinese people do not look much different from their ancestors.

Communes

We visited several communes in the countryside and found them to be very practical and functional units. A few members of our group were given permission to live in one of these communes for a few days, but unfortunately, in view of our limited stay in China, this wasn't possible.

An average commune has about 65,000 people, although there are larger and smaller communes. The people appear to get along with each other very well and are all hard working. There was no dishonesty involved in handling their finances. At most of the communes that we visited we were given reports on their financial situation and a breakdown of their income and expense. Since there are no taxes, they contribute a certain percentage of their agricultural products to the national food stockpile.

The communes are self-sufficient units, with their own local government, health care systems, and schools. They do receive help from the government in the form of surplus People's Liberation Army personnel who are sent to work on the farms. The government also helps with higher education of students from communes and takes seriously ill patients from commune hospitals into the big city hospitals for treatment.

Within a commune system, an individual Chinese farmer is happier than his ancestors were. He eats better, has more security and can look forward to a promising future for his children. Wherever we visited with the old farmers they told us of the hard days that they had experienced prior to Liberation when they were at the mercy of the landlords. Now they are secure and happy. In spite of the commune system, they are allowed to own small parts of land in their own back yards where they can grow vegetables or raise small animals for their personal use. If they make any money from these ventures, they may keep it and do not have to give it to the communal fund. They are also allowed to own their own houses.

Arts:

Since I am a collector of paintings and other art objects, I was interested in finding some examples of traditional Chinese art. The stores in Shanghai and Peking had quite a few of these old art works at reasonable prices. Nobody living in China seems to buy them.

Very few of the modern Chinese painters do any landscapes or abstract paintings. Most of their works are of a revolutionary nature. For the most part they were commissioned for state offices and institutions, but some of the less expensive ones are available for the citizens to buy. It was hard for me to believe that an artist, who is a creative individual, can be made to produce only politically oriented art. Although the Chinese craftsmen continue to manufacture art objects such as ivory carvings and snuff bottles for export, there is virtually no demand for such objects within China.

Literature:

I browsed through many bookstores during my visit, but saw only political and technical literature for sale in China. No foreign books or their Chinese translations are available. The large library of Western books at Peking University was closed for students, although we were allowed to examine it. I could find no novels written by contemporary Chinese writers and no translations of current foreign best-selling novels. The Chinese, however, have a great curiosity and hunger for reading and only recently some productions of ancient Chinese books, as well as some translations of Western books, were put on the market on a limited scale. They sold out as fast as they were delivered to the stores. There is strict control on books brought in by visitors. Chinese authorities see to it that visitors take all their books back with them when they leave the country.

Cultural Life and Entertainment:

I saw no night clubs or bars in China and there were very few movie houses and theatres. Most of the entertainment consists of revolutionary plays and movies. We were invited to quite a few of these—most of them dealt with the struggle of the Chinese against the Japanese occupation and with incidents that occurred during the War of Liberation. No foreign movies are shown in China, but they produce some excellent documentary films about nature. However, the entertainment I enjoyed most were the cultural gatherings where art performances were given by the children. Though these were also politically oriented, it was interesting to see young children with so much acting ability. But the best performances were in the Chinese circus.

We were treated as guests at all the performances we attended. Even when the theatre was full, the Chinese would stand up and make room for us. We were allowed to photograph and record the music. The Chinese greatly enjoy these performances and whole families go including the little children. Since there are no privately-owned TV sets, the theatre or movie is one of the few forms of entertainment.

Industry:

China is becoming an industrial nation. There are large factories in Shanghai and many other factories spread throughout the countryside. They manufacture virtually everything (except large jet transport planes) including their own jet fighter planes. Their automobiles are quite expensive. A good Chinese car costs around $5,000 to $6,000 but the high price is no problem since individuals are not allowed to own cars.

Most of the medical equipment manufactured in China, such as x-ray equipment, is very similar to the modern x-ray equipment in the West. It is even possible that they have duplicated Western machines. Some of the precision instruments, such as watches and cameras, are of very good quality and comparable to Western products, although much lower priced.

The Educational System:

The Chinese educational system has been greatly modified and simplified since Liberation. The emphasis is now on practice and not on theory. There is a tremendous amount of political indoctrination at all levels, from kindergarten to postgraduate work. It is impossible to make a sensible comparison with the educational system of the West. The Chinese children get a limited view of the world. They are only taught what the Chinese government feels is appropriate for them to know. In a Chinese classroom some countries are referred to as "friends" and others as "enemies." The children are well disciplined, but I think the education they are receiving will leave them with a lot to learn in terms of understanding and communicating with the rest of the nations of this world.

Education is free and available to all who are interested. While basic education is compulsory, a student is chosen for higher, specialized, technical education. This choice is not made on scholastic achievement but on political standing and with the recommendation of a person in the community. There are no examinations. After a student has completed his studies, he immediately starts practicing the profession for which he has been trained.

The Making of New Men in China:

It has been commented from time to time that Mao is attempting to remake the Chinese into a new form of superior being. It is difficult for me to give an opinion on this topic. The Chinese are certainly very disciplined and puritanical and if one were to use these as criteria of superiority they would rank very high. On the other hand, if one uses material progress or freedom as an individual for a measure, the Chinese rank low.

A true assessment of Chinese culture will remain impossible for some time to come, but two things are certain—it will have a significant impact on the West as we come in closer contact with China, and Chinese culture will be altered by its familiarity with our Western world.

Index